MANUAL OF DENTAL THERAPEUTICS

Manual of Dental Therapeutics

Raymond F. Zambito, D.D.S., Ed.D., M.B.A.
*Chairman, Department of Dentistry
Catholic Medical Center of Brooklyn and
    Queens, Inc.
Jamaica, New York
Former Professor, Oral and Maxillofacial
    Surgery and Anesthesiology
Fairleigh S. Dickinson, Jr. College of
    Dental Medicine
Fairleigh Dickinson University
Hackensack, New Jersey*

James J. Sciubba, D.M.D., Ph.D.
*Chairman, Department of Dentistry
Long Island Jewish Medical Center
New Hyde Park, New York
Professor of Oral Pathology
State University of New York at Stony
    Brook
School of Dental Medicine
Stony Brook, New York*

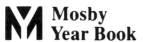
**Mosby
Year Book**

St. Louis   Baltimore   Boston   Chicago   London   Philadelphia   Sydney   Toronto

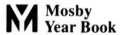

Mosby
Year Book

Dedicated to Publishing Excellence

Sponsoring Editor: Robert W. Reinhardt
Assistant Managing Editor, Text and Reference: George Mary Gardner
Production Project Coordinator: Carol A. Reynolds
Proofroom Manager: Barbara Kelly

Mosby–Year Book, Inc.
11830 Westline Industrial Drive
St. Louis, MO 63146

2   3   4   5   6   7   8   9   0 CLSE 95   94   93   92

Library of Congress Cataloging-in-Publication Data

Manual of dental therapeutics / [edited by] Raymond F. Zambito, James
   J. Sciubba.
        p.   cm.
   Includes bibliographical references and index.
   ISBN 0-8151-9895-7
   1. Mouth—Diseases.   2. Oral manifestations of general diseases.
   I. Zambito, Raymond F.   II. Sciubba, James J.
   [DNLM: 1. Mouth Diseases—therapy.   WU 166 M294]
   RK307.M36   1991
   617.5′2206—dc20   91-4834
   DNLM/DLC   CIP
   for Library of Congress

To our families and our residents, past and present, all of whom have helped us realize that success comes when preparation meets opportunity

CONTRIBUTORS

Anthony J. Casino, D.D.S.

Assistant Professor
Oral and Maxillofacial Surgery
State University of New York at
  Stony Brook
School of Dental Medicine
Stony Brook, New York
Chief, Oral and Maxillofacial
  Surgery
Northport Veterans
  Administration Medical Center
Northport, New York

Paul V. Crespi, D.D.S.

Assistant Professor
Pediatric Dentistry
State University of New York at
  Stony Brook
School of Dental Medicine
Stony Brook, New York
Chief, Division of Pediatric
  Dentistry
Schneider Children's Hospital
Long Island Jewish Medical
  Center
New Hyde Park, New York

Frederick A. Curro, D.M.D.,
Ph.D.

Vice President, Clinical Research
  and Pharmacology
Block Drug Company, Inc.
Jersey City, New Jersey
Attending, Department of
  Dentistry
St. Joseph's Hospital and
  Medical Center
Patterson, New Jersey

Paul D. Freedman, D.D.S.

Assistant Director
Section of Oral Pathology
Booth Memorial Medical Center
Director, Oral Pathology
  Laboratory, Inc.
Flushing, New York

Stanley M. Kerpel, D.D.S.

Adjunct Assistant Professor of
  Dentistry (Oral Pathology)
New York Medical College
Valhalla, New York
Attending in Dentistry and
  Pathology
Booth Memorial Medical Center
Flushing, New York

Gerard F. Koorbusch, D.D.S.,
M.B.A.

Assistant Professor
Director, Pre-Doctoral Oral and
  Maxillofacial Surgery
University of Iowa
College of Dentistry
Iowa City, Iowa

Daniel M. Laskin, D.D.S.,
M.S.

Professor and Chairman
Department of Oral and
  Maxillofacial Surgery
Medical College of Virginia
School of Dentistry
Richmond, Virginia

David A. Lederman, D.M.D.

Adjunct Associate Professor
Department of Pathology
Fairleigh S. Dickinson, Jr.
  College of Dental Medicine
Fairleigh Dickinson University
Hackensack, New Jersey
Past President (1989–1990)
American Academy of Oral
  Medicine

Harry Lumerman, D.D.S.

Clinical Professor
Oral Medicine and Oral
  Pathology
New York University College of
  Dentistry
New York, New York
Director, Oral Pathology
Booth Memorial Medical Center
Flushing, New York

Arthur Mashberg, D.D.S.

Chief, Oral and Maxillofacial
  Surgery
Deputy Chief, Cancer Center
Veterans Administration Medical
  Center
East Orange, New Jersey

Francis B. Olsen, D.D.S.,
M.P.A.

Assistant Professor of Dental
  Health
State University of New York at
  Stony Brook
School of Dental Medicine
Stony Brook, New York
Chief, Division of General
  Dentistry
Department of Dental Medicine
Long Island Jewish Medical
  Center
New Hyde Park, New York

Robert M. Peskin, D.D.S.

Clinical Assistant Professor of
  Dental Medicine
  (Anesthesiology)
State University of New York at
  Stony Brook
School of Dental Medicine
Stony Brook, New York
Section of Dental Anesthesiology
Department of Dental Medicine
Long Island Jewish Medical
  Center
New Hyde Park, New York

James J. Sciubba, D.M.D.,
Ph.D.

Professor of Oral Pathology
State University of New York at
  Stony Brook
School of Dental Medicine
Stony Brook, New York
Chairman, Department of Dental
  Medicine
Long Island Jewish Medical
  Center
New Hyde Park, New York

Lorraine B. Tesch, R.N., B.S.

Former Consultant, Division of
  Hospital Dentistry
Department of Oral and
  Maxillofacial Surgery and
  Anesthesiology
Fairleigh S. Dickinson, Jr.
  College of Dental Medicine
Fairleigh Dickinson University
Hackensack, New Jersey
Health Care Programs
  Consultant
Prudential Insurance Company
Roseland, New Jersey

Raymond F. Zambito, D.D.S.,
Ed.D., M.B.A.

Chairman, Department of
  Dentistry
Catholic Medical Center of
  Brooklyn and Queens, Inc.
Jamaica, New York
Former Professor, Oral and
  Maxillofacial Surgery and
  Anesthesiology
Fairleigh S. Dickinson, Jr.
  College of Dental Medicine
Fairleigh Dickinson University
Hackensack, New Jersey

FOREWORD

I am deeply honored to write the Foreword for *Manual of Dental Therapeutics,* which has arisen from needs perceived by two astute clinician/educators who have led a successful task in strengthening the medical/dental interface. This book is patterned after the highly acclaimed *Manual of Medical Therapeutics,* which has enjoyed a superb reputation with wide distribution among our medical and dental colleagues.

The *Manual of Dental Therapeutics* promises to be an invaluable asset of excellent quality for dental students, residents, and practicing dentists. Information in this text is essential to any practitioner caring for the oral health needs of today's society.

The authors have succinctly and cleverly brought together current topics that can be utilized by all those participating in the delivery of dental and oral health care. The text material is concise and easily readable. All chapters are treated in the same general format, focusing on presenting symptoms followed by differential diagnosis and the options for therapy, with consequent outcomes. The material presented covers a wide range of dental and orofacial problems, including infections, trauma, various types of lesions, and the medically compromised patient, to name but a few. This book is a significant addition to the library of all dental professionals, and will certainly provide the necessary knowledge to enable them to become better diagnosticians and providers of dental care.

Louis F. Rose, D.D.S., M.D.
Professor of Medicine and Surgery
Chief, Division of Dental Medicine
The Medical College of Pennsylvania
Professor of Periodontics
Chairman of Continuing Education
University of Pennsylvania
School of Dental Medicine
Philadelphia, Pennsylvania

PREFACE

The idea for this manual was initiated by long years of using the *Manual of Medical Therapeutics* during residency and hospital dentistry and oral/maxillofacial surgery practice. In addition, the experiences of residents over the years with the same manual strengthened the desire to produce such a manual for the clinical practice of general dentistry and its specialties.

Our purpose was further refined as we reviewed the times more defined diagnostic and management skills were needed. Thus this manual was developed to traverse the void dental clinicians, generalists, and specialists often find themselves in when addressing particular clinical situations. Such situations often arise when a patient presents with concomitant dental and general medical problems or with oral and head and neck conditions requiring that enhanced level of diagnostic and therapeutic acumen. Our goal was to fuse the diagnostic and therapeutic aspects of care against a background of applied basic science, including anatomy, microbiology, and pharmacology.

Our approach sought to eliminate the mechanical and empirical aspects of patient management. This was accomplished by applying rationale for clinical and therapeutic decisions based on various clinical paradigms. The various chapters of the manual attempt to assist the clinician in embracing and integrating a large array of current clinical findings in order to make a diagnosis and formulate a treatment plan. The perspective taken has been wide, to account for the majority of patients presenting in the outpatient setting. However, selected subjects and clinical situations cannot exclude inpatient management of patients with severe odontogenic infections, squamous cell carcinoma, certain medically compromising diseases, and odontogenic and salivary gland neoplasms.

The several clinicians chosen to assist in this endeavor come from all areas of clinical practice, research, and management. Most are seasoned clinicians with long histories of contributions to the profession. Several are new to the book writing world, while offering many years of expert clinical practice. All in all, we are pleased with the outcome of what appeared to be uncomplicated task when we started and turned out to be an endeavor of enterprise, creativity, and renewed vigor for the project and the need to integrate more and more the complexities of disease states with the ever more demanding need for knowledge.

Raymond F. Zambito, D.D.S., Ed.D., M.B.A.
James J. Sciubba, D.M.D., Ph.D.

CONTENTS

Patient Evaluation and Diagnosis

Anthony J. Casino

_____

Establishment of a diagnosis at the clinical or laboratory level mandates evaluation along several avenues. Delineation of local and systemic factors is necessary, and is accomplished by examination of the patient and formulation of a differential diagnosis and finally a definitive (working) diagnosis.

I. INFORMATION GATHERING
A. Chief complaint (CC)

The chief complaint is the specific reason for the patient's visit to the office or hospital. The chief complaint should be briefly recorded using the patient's own words, in quotation marks, when possible. An attempt should be made to have the patient identify the major problem, even if there seem to be several closely related complaints.

1

B. History of present illness (HPI)

The history of the present illness should provide the following information:

1. **Duration of signs and symptoms** (S&S) of chief complaint (acute or chronic).
2. **Concomitant symptoms:**
   a. **Pain** (quality and characteristics).
   b. **Dysfunction** of regional anatomic structures (e.g., trismus, dysphagia, xerostomia).
   c. **Systemic complaints** (e.g., fever, malaise, night sweats, dysfunction of other systems).
3. **Changes at site of complaint:**
   a. **Size:**
      (1) Increasing.
      (2) Decreasing.
   b. **Rate of change:**
      (1) Slow growth.
      (2) Rapid growth.
   c. **Color:**
      (1) Erythema.
      (2) Other color changes.
4. **Time when swelling or other symptoms noted:**
   a. Mealtime.
   b. Morning, evening, etc.
5. **Alterations of neural transmission:**
   a. Paresthesia.
   b. Anesthesia.
   c. Dysesthesia.
6. **Allergies:**
   a. Foods.
   b. Medications.
7. **Trauma:**
   a. Surgery.
   b. Accident.

C. Past medical/surgical history (PMH)

Factual information is elicited regarding any major health problems the patient has had. Determine whether the patient is a reliable historian, and obtain family corroboration if reliability is questionable.

D. Review of systems (ROS)

This comprehensive review is based on questions about symptomatic changes in various organ systems (e.g., respiratory, cardiovascular, gastrointestinal, hematologic, neurologic, genitourinary).

E. Physical examination (PE)

The components of a proper physical examination include (1) inspection, (2) palpation, and (3) percussion and auscultation.

1. Inspection

The clinical examination of facial swelling or other complaint begins with an accurate description (e.g., size, shape, consistency) and understanding of the anatomic region of the signs and symptoms; this information may provide the main clue to the diagnosis. The examination documents (a) anatomic location, (b) reaction to palpation, (c) texture and consistency, (d) relationship to adjacent tissues, and (e) dysfunction of anatomic structures.

a. Anatomic location:

(1) Face:

a. **Upper third:** infraorbital region to hairline.

b. **Middle third:** upper lip to infraorbital region.

c. **Lower third:** chin to upper lip.

(2) Neck:

a. **Anterior triangle:**

1. Digastric (submandibular) triangle.

2. Carotid triangle.

3. Submental triangle.

4. Muscular triangle.

b. **Posterior triangle:**

1. Occipital triangle.

2. Supraclavicular triangle.

(3) Lymph nodes:

a. **Head:**

1. Occipital.

2. Retroauricular.

3. Parotid.

4. Buccal (facial).

b. **Neck:**

1. Submandibular.

2. Submental.

3. Anterior cervical (superficial/deep).

       4. Posterior cervical (superficial/deep).

       5. Supraclavicular.

Lymphadenitis and metastatic carcinoma may present as lymph node swelling in the neck.

2. Palpation

Clinical information gained from palpation includes (1) texture, (2) temperature, (3) consistency, (4) tenderness, (5) relationship to adjacent tissues (e.g., fixed, movable), and (6) delineation.

3. Percussion and auscultation

Percussion and auscultation are rarely used in the clinical examination of facial swelling. Auscultation may be used if a mass is near the carotid artery, to differentiate a **bruit** from a pulsatile lesion, for example, an arteriovenous malformation.

F. Laboratory data (LABS)

Laboratory data include the results of (1) radiographic examination, (2) laboratory testing, and (3) tissue diagnostic techniques.

1. Radiographic examination

Radiographs **confirm** clinical findings and are performed **after** the clinical examination is completed.

a. Facial radiographs:

    (1) Skull series (posteroanterior [PA] and lateral).

    (2) Maxillary sinus (Waters view; open mouth and/or upright).

    (3) Submental vertex (zygomatic arch view).

    (4) Orbital radiographs (Reese view, tomograms).

    (5) Mandible series (PA and lateral oblique).

    (6) Towne projection.

    (7) Panoramic.

    (8) Occlusal.

    (9) Periapical.

    (10) Temporomandibular joint (TMJ) projection. Facial radiographs are useful in diagnosis of bony lesions and salivary stones (sialoliths), in detection of foreign bodies, and in evaluation of traumatic injuries and dental and jaw disease.

Computed tomography (CT) is excellent for evaluation of facial swelling and other head and neck lesions. The CT scan provides views of hard and soft tissues. The anatomy can be viewed in all planes of space and reference (coronal, axial, sagittal). Intravenously administered contrast material enhances soft tissue structures and blood vessels. Newer, more advanced units enable specific tissue densities to be compared with known tissues and lesions (e.g., muscle, lymph nodes, cysts, infection). Three-dimensional CT reconstruction also is possible on both flat films and skeletal model reproductions.

b. **Specialized radiologic studies:**
   (1) **Arteriography:** Used to differentiate vascular lesions and AV malformations.
   (2) **Magnetic resonance imaging (MRI):** Highly selective for soft tissues; can be reconstructed in all planes of space and is excellent for analyzing soft tissue masses, including internal derangements of the TMJ.
   (3) **Sialography:** Can be performed to diagnose some types of salivary gland disease (e.g., tumor, obstruction). Radiopaque dye is injected retrograde into the major salivary gland duct system via cannula, then plain films or CT is used to image the gland. Fluoroscopy is used to videotape sialography.
   (4) **Ultrasound:** An excellent means of evaluating facial and neck masses. Images obtained offer good delineation of solid tumor masses from fluid-filled infectious or cystic lesions.
   (5) **Nuclear medicine scanning:** Radionuclide imaging of swelling and masses in the head and neck is useful in determining cellular activity within the lesion. Offers a differential diagnosis in many specific lesions (e.g., thyroid neoplasia, bone tumor, certain types of salivary gland disease).

2. **Laboratory testing**
   a. **Complete blood cell count:**
      (1) White blood cell count.
      (2) Red blood cell count.
      (3) Hemoglobin.
      (4) Hematocrit.
      (5) Red blood cell indices.
      (6) White blood cell differential.
      (7) Peripheral blood cell morphology.
   b. **Serum chemistry (SMAC).**
   c. **Serology (virology):**
      (1) Monospot (infectious mononucleosis).
      (2) Serum heterophile.
      (3) Epstein-Barr virus titer.
      (4) Cytomegalovirus titer.
      (5) *Toxoplasma* titer.
      (6) Hepatitis.
      (7) Rubella.
      (8) Human immunodeficiency virus (HIV).
   d. **Specialized testing:**
      (1) Purified protein derivative (PPD) tuberculin skin test.
      (2) Kviem test (sarcoidosis).
      (3) Antinuclear antibodies.
   e. **Erythrocyte sedimentation rate (ESR).**
3. **Tissue diagnostic techniques (DX)**
   Procurement of representative tissue formulates the basis of a specific diagnosis. In addition to host tissue, in the form of a biopsy specimen, culture and sensitivity testing may be considered an analogous technique in the case of infectious disease.
   a. **Biopsy:**
      Several biopsy techniques have evolved. The traditional techniques remain incisional and excisional biopsy. In incisional biopsy a portion of a lesion or mass is removed for histologic examination. This technique usually is used in large lesions, with the goal of supplying adequate representative material to the pathologist. In excisional biopsy an entire lesion or mass is removed. This usually is the treatment of choice in small lesions, and generally is curative.

Other forms of biopsy include needle biopsy and aspiration biopsy. The more traditional needle biopsy (true cut) yields a core or plug of tissue for analysis; fine-needle aspiration provides the pathologist with individual cells or small clusters of cells for analysis. True aspiration biopsy is useful in analysis of suspected fluid-filled masses or lesions. The aspirate itself may be analyzed by microbiologic, cytologic, or biochemical means, among others. This technique should be attempted with a large-guage needle (18 guage or larger) for ease of aspiration, particularly if the content of the mass or lesion is viscous. Exfoliative cytology smear techniques can be used for surface lesions.

   b. **Culture and sensitivity testing:**
   The microbiologic identification process may be required for lesions for processes caused by infection. A Gram stain is routinely performed on all purulent aspirations and lesion specimens of suspected infectious cause. Such specimens also are submitted for culture and sensitivity testing. Culture includes techniques of acquisition for anaerobic and aerobic organisms. Special transport media are available for these techniques. Suspected fungal infections require special media and labeling. If sufficient quantity of aspirate is available, the sealed syringe may be sent for microbiologic processing.

G. **Differential diagnosis**
   Subsequent to gathering the data base, a differential diagnosis is established. The correlation matches a selection from the data base with a listing of possible causes of the chief complaint. Often tissue diagnostic techniques are the final step in the task of relating the chief complaint to a diagnosis. The results are then integrated into a working diagnosis and treatment plan.

BIBLIOGRAPHY

Halstead CL, Blozis CG, Drinan AJ, et al: *Physical Evaluation of the Dental Patient*. St Louis, CV Mosby, 1982.

Macklis RM, Mendelsohn ME, Mudge GH Jr: *Manual of Introductory Clinical Medicine: A Student-to-Student Guide.* Boston, Little, Brown, 1986.

Orland MJ, Saltman RJ (eds): *Manual of Medical Therapeutics,* ed 25. Boston, Little, Brown, 1987.

Chapter 2 _____

Odontogenic Infections

Raymond F. Zambito

_____

I. BACTERIAL INFORMATION

Bacterial information on infective agents as they relate to odontogenic infections includes the following:
1. The normal flora of the oral cavity are the usual causative agents in odontogenic infections.

9

2. Odontogenic infections are caused mainly by multiple bacteria. Rarely is one bacteria responsible for the infection, and laboratory reports may reveal as many as five species present in an infection.
3. Usual bacteria involved are aerobic gram-positive cocci, anaerobic gram-positive cocci, and anaerobic gram-negative rods.
4. Laboratory results identify a predominance of anaerobic bacteria, although as many as 60% of infections are mixed.
5. The mix of aerobic and anaerobic, gram-positive and gram-negtive species is estimated as:
   a. Aerobic: *Streptococcus,* 70%; *Staphylococcus,* 6%.
   b. Anaerobic: *Peptostreptococcus, Streptococcus,* and *Peptococcus,* 33%.
   c. Gram-positive rods, 15%.
   d. Gram-negative rods: *Bacteroides* group, about 34%; *Fusobacterium,* 13%.
6. Although multiple bacteria may be present, the actual progress of the infective process depends on the symbiotic relationship of these bacteria; several may aid each other, with varying predominance, depending on the time lapse of the infective process.

II. USE OF ANTIMICROBIALS

The use of antibiotics in every infective process is not indicated and should not be considered an absolute. Determinants for antibiotic as well as surgical therapy include:

1. Seriousness of the infective process, including the speed with which the infection is spreading (hours rather than days). Diffuse cellulitis and evidence of soft tissue intraoral swelling generally requires antibiotic therapy with surgical drainage.
2. Previous or current history of immunocompromise or diminished host defense. These generally require medical support with antibiotics.
3. Evidence of extraoral swelling. This is indicative of diffuse spread into fascial spaces and requires antibiotic therapy.

The clinical signs of *Staphylococcus* and *Streptococcus* involvement are described in Table 2–1.

The three stages (with clinical differences) in an infective process are *inflammation, cellulitis,* and *abscess formation.* Inflammation is the earliest clinical sign of injury to tissue. Classic signs are calor (heat), dolor (pain), rubor (redness), and tumor (swelling). This first stage of the infective process can last 3 to 5 days.

The process may progress to cellulitis. Cellulitis is characterized by rapid onset or acute manifestation, and the area of involvement is large compared with the cause (e.g., a tooth), with diffuse borders that may be raised or indurated, red or scarlet in comparison with the surrounding tissues, with no evidence of pus formation; pain is usually an important factor. The major bacteria are streptococcus organisms.

The process from inflammation to abscess is usually slower, the involved area is less painful, with well-circumscribed borders, and purulent material within the borders is identified via palpation. It is usually less aggressive and of longer duration.

Radiographic interpretation of periapical lesions can be misleading. On intraoral radiographs, changes at the apex of a tooth may be misdiagnosed as an abscess. Evidence of a periapical rarefaction (change in apical density) indicates a dynamic pro-

TABLE 2–1.
Comparison of *Staphylococcus* and *Streptococcus*

	Staphylococcus	*Streptococcus*
Discovered	1880	1880
Found in	Boils, abscesses	Throat, skin, as a parasite
Emits toxins	Yes	Yes
Erythrogenic factor	No	Yes
Occludes lymph channels	In 8–12 hours	In 36–72 hours
Elaborates hyaluronidase	No	Yes
Spreads via	Ducts, arteries, direct extension	Lymph channels, direct extension
Complications	Mostly local, and septicemia	Local, plus carditis, nephritis, rheumatic fever, rheumatic heart disease, orchitis, septicemia

cess. The end point may be chronic inflammation resulting in granuloma or cyst formation. The radiolucent area may also be the result of previous apical surgery where new bone has not filled in the defect. For the diagnosis of abscess, periapical radiolucency must be accompanied by clinical signs of infection, namely, pain, swelling, tenderness to touch or percussion, and soft tissue involvement. A fistula indicates the presence of chronic infection.

III. MICROFLORA OF ORAL CAVITY

The oral cavity is essentially sterile at birth. However, it can retain nutritional components such as carbohydrates, proteins, lipids, and amino acids. Microorganisms appear soon after birth, as a result of normal delivery via the vaginal canal, breast-feeding, and holding and handling the baby. Species of *Streptococcus, Staphylococcus, Neisseria,* and *Veillonella* appear within a few days of birth. Species not present at this time are the obligate anaerobic bacteria, and appear as teeth erupt secondary to gingival crevice formation and the development of plaque that supports anaerobes.

As teeth erupt, *Actinomyces, Bacteroides, Fusobacterium,* and *Leptotrichia* become normal flora components. In addition, spirochetes, fusiform bacilli, and *Vibrio* increase in number. *Bacteroides melaninogenicus* and spirochetes take up permanent status in the oral cavity during puberty; hormonal change is considered responsible. *Streptococcus mutans* and *Streptococcus sanguis* arrive with the teeth, and are capable of attaching directly to enamel and other hard surfaces. It appears that the ability of bacteria to adhere to surfaces is a major determining factor in their continued existence in the oral cavity; this phenomena occurs at other anatomic sites as well.

Specific microorganisms are found in specific places in the oral cavity. The microflora of the gingival crevices are specific to it, as are bacteria that colonize the tongue, and dental plaque.

None of the approximately 300 species of bacteria in the oral cavity exist in isolation. Codependence and interdependence are essential, in many cases, for survival, and thus for pathologic conditions such as infection to occur.

IV. ANTIBIOTIC SUSCEPTIBILITY TESTING

Methods for determining antibiotic susceptibility include (1) disk agar diffusion, (2) quantitative dilution methods, and (3) automated methods. The disk agar method is the most commonly used, although the quantitative dilution methods are becoming more popular in the United States. Laboratories may use both disk agar and quantitative dilution for effective testing. Testing for slow-growing, nutritionally and environmentally restrictive organisms, such as *Haemophilus influenzae, Neisseria gonorrhoeae, Bacteroides fragilis,* and other anaerobes, require the dilution methods.

The common antibiogram used today to identify susceptibility has four categories:

Group 1: Organisms with a high degree of susceptibility to normal/usual doses of antibiotic, called "susceptible"

Group 2: Organisms requiring higher doses of antibiotics, even up to the limits of toxicity

Group 3: Organisms with a degree of susceptibility requiring concentration of the antibiotic at the local site

Group 4: Organisms with a degree of both susceptibility and resistance giving a questionable response, termed "resistant"

Anaerobic susceptibility testing requires special consideration of the method to be used. The antibiotics generally recommended for anaerobe testing are cefoxitin, chloramphenicol, clindamycin, moxalactam, carbenicillin (ticarcillin or piperacillin), and metronidazole. Penicillin is considered if there is concern for the presence of *Clostridium.*

Susceptibility tests evaluate given concentrations of the antibiotic on the growth of a known number of bacteria. All bacteria, both aerobes and anaerobes, can exhibit a wide range of growth characteristics. The rapid disk susceptibility test, the most widely used, is standardized for rapidly growing, aerobic, and facultative anaerobic bacteria. This test relies on the value given to the zone of inhibition. In the rapid broth dilution method a specific amount of the collected material to be tested is put into a series of dilutions of the antimicrobial. It usually takes

18 hours by this method to identify the minimal inhibitory concentration (MIC), that is, the lowest concentration of the antimicrobial that will inhibit visible growth of the organism.

The rapid assay for β-lactamase, a rapid discovery test, is used to assess the resistance to penicillin. *N. gonorrhoeae, H. influenzae,* and *Staphylococcus aureas* are of especial interest as penicillin-resistant organisms.

V. LABORATORY DIAGNOSIS

Why consider susceptibility testing when most patients with odontogenic infections receive empirical therapy? The reasons include:

1. The patient receives the benefit of knowing the actual microbe involved.
2. Reduction in energy, time, and cost follows if the infection does not respond to empirical therapy.
3. Therapy is determined on hard evidence specific to the patient's problem.
4. The information contributes to the education of the clinician for future reference in similar cases.
5. Recommendations for preventive therapy can be developed from the data obtained.

Selective testing and perhaps special collection and isolation techniques may be required for isolation of disease-producing organisms taken from areas that normally harbor many species of flora, such as the oropharynx, oral cavity, gastrointestinal tract, and vagina. In addition, certain conditions may affect survival of organisms after collection and transportation. Thus knowledge of the considered organism's requirements will obviate repeated testing. The clinician must be aware of the needs of the laboratory, and specifically, whether aerobic or anaerobic culture media and testing are required for a definitive diagnosis. The more rapidly the specimen is delivered to the laboratory after collection the more reliable will be the result. It is recommended that polyester fiber swabs be used to collect specimens, because cotton swabs may contain lipoproteins that can inhibit certain bacteria. Transport medium is essential when the collected material cannot be immediately delivered to the laboratory. Transport media are designed to protect the organism from drying out or dying, and also inhibit overgrowth of contaminant organisms.

Gram stain is a reliable and quick method for identifying bacteria or fungi; however, lack of familiarity with the procedure may lead to inaccurate interpretation. Other stains used for rapid identification include acid-fast stains and fluorescein-tagged antibodies. The latter are especially useful for identifying group A β-hemolytic streptococci.

The clinician is advised to visit a laboratory of choice to discuss the various methods used to assist in the identification of microorganisms and susceptibility testing for aerobic and anaerobic bacteria.

VI. ODONTOGENIC INFECTIONS

Odontogenic infections, their localization and spread are controlled by the bony structures in which the teeth are embedded, the muscle attachments, and the fascial layers that surround the muscular tissues. Knowledge of the location of the apex of the tooth and its relationship to muscular attachments and muscular functions as well as the relationship of the apex to cortical bone and to fascial spaces is essential to clinical diagnosis. The reader is directed to a textbook of dental anatomy for further identification of these relationships as they are explained in the presentation that follows.

A. Pulpal Pain

Patients have a history of intermittent pain, which may present variably over time. Generally pulpal pain is caused by a noxious stimulus, such as heat, cold, or other change in the environment of the tooth. The patient complains of pain that can run the gamut from nuisance to throbbing pain that is not relieved by home therapy. In addition, as the inflammatory process continues, pain may be increased by thermal changes or may be intensified with heat and relieved by cold. Appropriate clinical examination with instruments and with bimanual palpation assists in identifying the offending tooth or teeth. Radiographs of the area may identify caries in a clinically appearing virginal tooth, caries under a filling, or a defect in either the enamel or the cementum, which affects the dentin and thus the pulp. The options for therapy include relief of pain with a local anesthetic in preparation for removal of the caries (if that is the source), elimination of an occlusal prematurity, sedation of exposed pulp that is still vital, or inception of endodontic therapy. The patient will require an analgesic, preferably aspirin or acetaminophen or other agent the patient prefers and has taken for headache or other minor pain; generally narcotic analgesics are not required for relief of pulpal pain.

B. Periapical and Periodontal Abscess

The patient may present with tenderness at the apex (identified clinically via mild swelling), which indicates that an inflammatory exudate has penetrated the cancellous and compact bone and expanded the periosteal structure, resulting in firm but tender swelling. Radiographs may or may not demonstrate periapical disease; however, they may reveal periodontal membrane thickening. Therapy may be endodontic or extraction.

Periapical abscess is characterized by swelling in the mucobuccal fold area that distorts the normal tissue architecture, indicating that the periapical infective process has passed through the bony structures, through the periosteum, and into soft tissues. The swelling is soft and may be exquisitely tender, with a thinned tissue center (pointing) more tender to the touch than the immediate surrounding tissues. The swelling is discrete, the tissue reddened and well demarcated. Therapy includes local incision for drainage of the abscess material. A specimen for routine culture and sensitivity studies may be taken at this time. Prescription of antibiotic therapy depends on the clinical presentation of the infective process and the clinical estimate of whether the process is in the ascendency or is quiescent. The clinician should look for elevated temperature ($>100°$ F orally), indicative of fever, and presence of acutely tender lymph nodes. Not all abscesses of the dentoalveolar structures require antibiotic therapy; all probably require surgical incision and drainage. Clinically, a pungent odor and gas escaping from a root canal signal anaerobic bacterial infection. Acceptable drainage through the tooth root canal is questionable, especially via a mandibular tooth. Generally the purulent material is too viscous to flow through the apex; thus drainage is limited.

Recognition of indications of spread beyond the area of the affected tooth (teeth) is essential to determination of the aggressiveness of therapy to be delivered. These indicators include swelling well beyond the site of initial infection, extraoral swelling not in keeping with expected spread of infection, trismus or guarding by the patient, difficulty in swallowing, infraorbital or periorbital swelling, loss of intraoral normal architecture of the soft palate and adjacent tissues, and swelling of the neck. Odontogenic infections generally spread by following the path of least resistance (e.g., apex proximity to cortical bone, muscle attachments deflecting infectious materials).

C. Pericoronitis

The patient presents with an erupting tooth, generally a molar, where the pericoronal tissues will not permit the tooth to completely erupt into the oral cavity. The tissues may surround part or all of the coronal and occlusal portion of the tooth, presenting a tissue impediment to appropriate occlusion with an opposing tooth. This occurs when soft tissue over the occlusal surface is traumatized by chewing or by the opposing tooth. The area is edematous, raised, red, and very tender to palpation and manipulation. The patient may complain of dysphagia and trismus. Radiographs may be difficult to obtain, and generally do not lend additional information for the diagnosis. The clinical presentation is generally sufficient to allow a diagnosis that is accurate and for which therapy is reasonably clear. Irrigation of the area is required to cleanse the pockets around the soft tisue structures surrounding the unerupted tooth. Patients should receive antibiotic coverage if there is fever (temperature >100° F orally), a clinical impression that the inflammation or infective process is in the ascendency and is of recent onset (i.e., 24 to 48 hours). Occlusion is checked to be certain that an opposing tooth is not exacerbating the problem. The patient is instructed to irrigate the area with warm saline solution or chlorhexidine *every hour* to reduce the inflammatory process as quickly as possible, and to ingest a soft diet. When the inflammatory stage has passed and the tissues return to normal, the pericoronal tissues are excised if space and local anatomy permit proper eruption of the tooth, or the tooth is extracted if eruption into a normal occlusal pattern is unlikely.

D. Canine Space Infection

The patient presents with swelling of the lateral alar area and puffiness under the eye. The skin may show a localized area of redness and edema and tenderness over the canine area. The process may be identified with the cuspid or the first bicuspid. The mucobuccal fold may not have lost its architecture, and the affected tooth (usually a bicuspid) is sensitive to percussion and to manipulation. A radiograph may or may not demonstrate periapical rarefaction. However, bimanual palpation of the area will give an indication of fluid contained within rigid confines over the periapical area. Anatomically, the canine space infection occurs between the levator anguli oris and the medial head of the levator labii superioris muscle. An infective process leaves the apex of the bicuspid or cuspid, erodes through the thin cortical plate, passes through the periosteum, and localizes between these two muscles rather than in a subperiosteal location, pushing the mucogingival tissue aside. If the origin of the infection is within the pulpal tissues, endodontic therapy is required. An incision and drainage ordinarily suffice for the release of purulent fluid from the area, provided the anatomic site is recognized to be between the muscles identified. Culture and sensitivity of the drainage definitely aids in prescribing the most effective antibiotic. A Gram stain will clarify the bacteria quickly. Mild over-the-counter analgesics are sufficient for pain relief.

E. Submental Space Infection

The patient presents with swelling under the chin and leading toward the trachea, well confined between the anterior bellies of the digastric muscles and generally the result of involvement of mandibular anterior teeth. Either periapical or periodontal infection as well as trauma to the area may have caused apical transfer of fluids and bacteria from the apex of the tooth into the submental structures. The submental space is bounded superiorly by the genioglossus muscle, inferiorly by the geniohyoid muscle, and laterally by the anterior bellies of the digastric muscles. There may be some edema of the floor of the mouth. Pain, induration, and tenderness are present. Radiographs usually identify the offending tooth (teeth). These patients often require antibiotic therapy, as well as extraoral incision to provide dependent drainage. Intraoral incision and exploration do not provide dependent drainage. Analgesics are in order.

F. Submandibular Space Infection

The submandibular space lies between the posterior belly of the digastric muscle as the posterior terminus and the anterior belly of the digastric as the forward portion; the mylohyoid muscle forms its roof. The inferior border of the mandible and the soft tissues of the side of the neck make up the lateral portion. The hyoid bone is the inferior border. Infections in this area usually originate in mandibular second or third molars, where the mylohyoid muscle crosses the apices of the mandibular teeth in its movement posterosuperiorly. Infective processes in the mandibular molars are close to the lingual cortex as the teeth move distally; thus inflammatory and infective processes erode easily through the lingual cortex into the submandibular space. Identifying the involved tooth (teeth) or periodontal structures requires careful clinical examination as well as radiographic survey. Extraoral incision and drainage of the submandibular space are necessary, because adequate superior drainage cannot be obtained intraorally. Such infective involvement of a fascial space requires adequate antibiotic therapy. Acute infection of this space may require that the patient be hospitalized. Penicillin G given intravenously is the drug of choice in nonallergic patients.

G. Floor of Mouth/Sublingual Space Infection

This space lies between the mylohyoid muscle sling inferiorly, and anteroposteriorly by the mucosa of the floor of the mouth. Access to the floor of the mouth/sublingual space is via all teeth from the incisors to the first molar, because the apices of these teeth are above the mylohyoid muscle attachment as it moves posteriorly and superiorly along the medial border of the mandible. Clinical examination, evidence of caries, periodontal disease, and radiographic support of the findings generally identify the involved tooth. Elevation of the floor of the mouth and tongue usually follows such invasion of the floor/sublingual space. There is anatomic access to the submandibular, submental, and lateral pharyngeal spaces, and involvement of these spaces is a potential complication. Incision and drainage of the floor of the mouth/sublingual space, necessary if the area in question is fluctuant, are carried out close to the mucogingival fold, that is, as close to the medial surface of the mandible as possible. This intervention avoids interrupting Wharton's duct or the lingual nerve.

H. Buccinator Space Infection

The buccinator space is contained between the buccinator muscle and the superficial fascia of the skin. The buccinator muscle is attached superiorly along the length of the maxilla from the cuspid posteriorly, and is inferiorly attached to the lateral surface of the mandible. An infective process in the maxillary bicuspids and first molar area can extend over the superior attachment of the buccinator muscle and into the fascial space between the muscle and the layer of skin, platysma, and superficial fascia. Occasionally infection can originate in a mandibular molar. The clinical presentation is that of a person blowing out his or her cheek. Trismus is minimal, and can assist in distinguishing a buccinator infection from a submasseteric infection. Once the diagnosis has been made and bimanual palpation identifies fluid within the buccinator space, incision for drainage is appropriate, and is performed in the mandibular mucobuccal fold to create dependent drainage. Drainage above the involved tooth (teeth) in the maxilla does not establish dependent drainage. Radiographs of the tooth (teeth) confirm the diagnosis. The use of antibiotic therapy is a clinical judgment. Analgesics are generally in order. Extraoral incision and drainage are avoided as the approach of first choice.

I. Pterygomandibular Space Infection

The pterygomandibular space is contained by the medial surface of the ramus, with the internal pterygoid muscle as the medial border and the pterygomandibular raphe as the anterior border (the fibrous connection between the buccinator muscle and the superior constrictor muscle); the posterior border is the deep lobe of the parotid gland. This space is clinically and therapeutically entered by inferior alveolar injection. Infective processes in this area can result from pericoronal infections around third molars. Infection can also be introduced via inferior alveolar injection if a hematoma forms or if infective material is carried into the pterygomandibular space with the needle. The clinical presentation may include pain, trismus, dysphagia, and tenderness. The patient generally is unable to open the mouth more than one finger width or guards against opening wider, because palpating the area causes pain. A bulge appears in the area of the peritonsillar structures, indicating that fluid in the area has deflected the internal pterygoid muscle medially. Incision and placement of a tube for drainage is in order, and is usually performed with the patient under general anesthesia. Surgical entry can be made at the raphe or just lateral to it. Intravenous antibiotics and analgesics are in order, as well as oral lavage with warm saline solution.

J. Infratemporal Space Infection

The infratemporal space is contained between the posterior border of the maxilla, the lateral plate of the sphenoid bone posteriorly, and mediolaterally by the zygomatic arch. Infective processes in this area generally result from trauma to posterior maxillary teeth, surgical removal of a maxillary second or third molar, or injection into the superior alveolar nerve. Patients present with trismus, and are lethargic and very tired. There generally is bulging of the tissues immediately above and below the zygomatic arch, giving the external impression of a dumbbell. The infratemporal and temporal spaces are interconnected, and it is not unusual for both spaces to be involved with the same infection. Surgical intervention means entering the space via the posterior maxilla. Antibiotics and culture and sensitivity are in order. Generally patients require hospitalization and aggressive treatment. Extension of infection from the infratemporal space to the cavernous sinus and orbit can occur.

K. Submasseteric Space Infection

The submasseteric space is bounded by the masseter muscle laterally, by the lateral border of the ramus medially, the buccinator muscle anteriorly, and the parotid gland posteriorly. Entrance of infection into this area may result from an infective process in a first, second, or third molar. The patient presents with trismus, marked swelling and tenderness of the masseteric area, and inability to open the mouth more than one finger width. The condition can be acute or chronic. Surgical intervention can be intraoral or extraoral. The extraoral approach is preferred because it offers better dependent drainage. Antibiotics and analgesics in the acute stage are in order. Chronic submasseteric abscess (present for 1 to 2 weeks) usually improves after incision and drainage.

L. Ludwig's Angina

For a diagnosis of Ludwig's angina the submandibular spaces bilaterally and the submental space must be involved. von Ludwig in 1836 originally described a swelling that killed 60% of the patients in 10 to 14 days. Today Ludwig's angina can cause asphyxiation within 24 hours, generally due to reaction of the tissues to the invading bacteria, usually *Streptococcus*. The major cause of Ludwig's angina is odontogenic, followed by trauma. The process begins in one of the submandibular spaces and easily spreads to the opposite submandibular space and the submental space, guided by the fascial layers, which offer ease of movement in circular and superoinferior directions because there are no barriers to prevent such extension. Therapy consists of hospitalization, airway protection, and aggressive surgical and antibiotic therapy.

M. Lateral Pharyngeal Space Infection

Infections of the lateral pharyngeal space generally are secondary to direct spread from contiguous structures. Sources include dental infections, chronic tonsillitis, and infection of the parotid gland. The anatomy of the space is variously identified as an inverted cone or triangle, with the base formed by the base of the skull and the apex by the hyoid bone. The space is bounded by the visceral layer of the deep cervical fascia that covers the superior pharyngeal constrictor muscle. On its lateral side the space is bounded by the fascia that covers the pterygoid muscles and the parotid gland. Communication exists with the submandibular, parotid and retropharyngeal spaces, which offer direct access to and from the lateral pharyngeal space. When the space is involved secondary to a dental infection, there is swelling that bulges toward the midline, often accompanied by fever, dysphagia, trismus, and deviation of the soft palate. There may be extraoral swelling at the angle of the mandible. This infection usually is not an isolated event but is noted in conjunction with multiple fascial space infections of the head and neck. Therapy includes aggressive intravenous antibiotic therapy and surgical drainage. These infections are generally life threatening, and must be identified quickly and treated immediately if the patient is to recover with minimal scarring or loss of function. Although drainage can usually be accomplished by intraoral intervention, the classic approach is extraoral incision in the neck. Airway management in the presence of lateral pharyngeal space infection may require tracheostomy if appropriate intubation is not feasible.

N. Retropharyngeal Space Infection

The retropharyngeal space often is involved as part of a pan-space infection of the potential spaces in the affected side of the patient's face and head. The space itself is made up of loose connective tissue that lies behind the pharynx, between the superior pharyngeal constrictor muscle and the alar layer of the prevertebral fascia. It extends from the base of the skull to the level of the tracheal bifurcation, usually at C-7 and T-1. Infections of this area are serious because of the potential for fatal spread into the mediastinum, which can be a route of spread to the diaphragm. Involvement of this space by orofacial or dentofacial infections may be diagnosed with lateral soft tissue radiographs, which demonstrate widening of the retropharyngeal space, or by computed tomography. Treatment of retropharyngeal space infection is by intraoral or cervical incision and drainage. The patient must be closely observed for spread of infection to the mediastinum. Aggressive medical and surgical therapy is required, generally with a multidisciplinary team approach.

BIBLIOGRAPHY

Hollinshead WH: *Anatomy for Surgeons,* vol 1, *The Head and Neck.* New York, Hoeber-Harper, 1960.

Manual on Medical Therapeutics, ed 25. Boston, Little, Brown, 1987.

Neu HC: *Antimicrobial Prescribing.* Princeton, NJ, Antimicrobial Prescribing, 1979.

Newman MG, Goodman AD: *Guide to Antibiotic Use in Dental Practice.* Chicago, Quintessence Publishing Co, 1984.

Peterson LJ, Ellis E III, Hupp JR, et al: *Contemporary Oral and Maxillofacial Surgery.* St Louis, CV Mosby Co, 1988.

Tiecke RW, Stuteville OH, Calandra JC: *Pathologic Physiology of Oral Disease.* St Louis, CV Mosby Co, 1959.

Topazian RG, Goldberg MH: *Management of Infections of the Oral and Maxillofacial Regions,* ed 2. Philadelphia, WB Saunders, 1987.

Zambito RF, Cleri DJ: *Immunology and Infectious Diseases of the Mouth, Head, and Neck.* St Louis, Mosby–Year Book, 1991.

Dentoalveolar Trauma

Paul V. Crespi

———————————

Dentoalveolar injury is a frequent and unpredictable occurrence with long-term and short-term physiologic and psychologic implications. It may be an isolated phenomenon, but often is associated with concomitant craniofacial injuries. Management of these injuries requires a systematic approach followed by a thoughtfully planned sequential treatment course.

The majority of dentoalveolar injuries involve the anterior teeth, because of their prominent position. Patients with maxillary anterior protrusion (class II malocclusion) or anterior dental procumbency secondary to unfavorable finger and sucking habits are predisposed to injury. The peak incidence of trauma to the primary dentition is between ages 1½ and 3 years. Subluxation, luxation, and avulsion of teeth are the most frequent injuries. By age 7 years more than 20% of girls and 30% of boys have sustained an injury to the dentoalveolar complex, dramatically highlighting the prevalence of this phenomena. In mixed dentition, a marked increase in traumatic dental injuries has been reported for boys 8 to 10 years of age. The majority of permanent tooth injuries are coronal fractures; less common permanent tooth injuries include concussion, luxation or subluxation, root fracture, dental avulsion, and alveolar fracture with associated soft tissue lacerations. These injuries to teeth and supporting structures can be defined as follows:

1. **Crown craze, or crack:** Horizontal or vertical crack or incomplete fracture of enamel without loss of tooth structure.
2. **Crown fracture:**
   a. May be confined to enamel or include dentin with or without pulp involvement. May be horizontal, vertical, or oblique, involving the mesioincisal or distoincisal line angles.
   b. **Ellis classification:**
   Class I: simple fracture of crown, involving little or no dentin.
   Class II: extensive fracture of crown, involving considerable dentin but not dental pulp.
   Class III: extensive fracture of crown with exposure of dental pulp.
   Class IV: loss of entire crown.
3. **Root fracture:** Horizontal or vertical fracture of the root involving the apical, middle, or cervical third.
4. **Concussion injury:** Injury to a tooth resulting in sensitivity of the tooth to touch or percussion but without any mobility or displacement.
5. **Subluxation:** Injury to tooth and supporting alveolus resulting in palpable tooth mobility without clinically discernible displacement.
6. **Luxation:** Tooth displacement in any plane, with concomitant alveolar bone damage.

    a. **Intrusion:** impaction of tooth into socket.

    b. **Extrusion:** partial displacement of tooth from socket.

    c. **Labial luxation:** buccal displacement of tooth.

    d. **Lingual luxation:** displacement of tooth toward palate or tongue.

    e. **Lateral luxation:** mesial or distal displacement of tooth.

7. **Avulsion:** Complete exarticulation of tooth from dental alveolus.

8. **Alveolar fracture:** Any fracture of alveolar bone as a component of luxated and subluxated dental injuries and dental avulsions. Segmental alveolar fractures result when a segment of alveolar bone, including teeth, is fractured in unison but the alveolar socket remains intact.

A dentoalveolar injury can be a tragic, traumatic episode, often with lifelong implications. It is generally the first serious injury sustained by a child, and produces family panic and undue emotional stress. The prognosis hinges on prompt, well-directed acute care management and follow-up therapy. Potential complications and untoward sequelae are considered and anticipated. Long-term treatment courses are expected, and include interim temporary measures for functional and esthetic considerations pending completion of the final restoration. Documentation of etiologic factors, existing conditions, and prognosis, plus good patient and family communication are essential. Diagnosis and predicted course of therapy are carefully discussed, including the prognosis for all procedures planned.

I. GENERAL CONSIDERATIONS

A. History

The past medical history emphasizes presence of bleeding diatheses, positive cardiac history, existence of allergies, current medications, history of immunocompromise, and immunization status, particularly for tetanus (Table 3–1). Patients with significant soft tissue wounds who have not been vaccinated should receive tetanus toxoid and human tetanus immune globulin immediately. Previously immunized patients are given a

TABLE 3–1.

Guide to Tetanus Prophylaxis in Wound Management*

History of Tetanus Immunization	Clean, Minor Wounds		All Other Wounds	
	TD	TIG	TD	TIG
Uncertain	Yes	No	Yes	Yes
0–1	Yes	No	Yes	Yes
2	Yes	No	Yes	No†
≥3	No‡	No	No§	No

*From American Academy of Pediatrics: *Report of the Committee on Infectious Disease,* ed 19. Elk Grove Village, Ill, The Academy, 1982, p 262. Used by permission.
†Unless wound is more than 24 hours old.
‡Unless more than 10 years since last dose.
§Unless more than 5 years since last dose.
TD = tetanus and diphtheria [toxoid]; TIG = tetanus immune globulin.

booster dose of tetanus toxoid if they have not received one in 5 to 10 years. Patients with a history of appropriate immunization and who have had a booster within 5 years of the traumatic episode require no additional tetanus therapy.

The dental history details the episode and includes the medical and legal considerations of the traumatic injury. A descriptive narrative regarding the cause of the accident, including geographic location and time of occurrence, is essential. The patient, if capable, is questioned about the presence of injuries beyond the oral and paraoral regions. Child abuse is not to be ruled out. The presence of disorientation, amnesia, loss of consciousness, or nausea and vomiting is documented. Neurologic symptoms necessitate medical evaluation and clearance before treatment is initiated.

B. Clinical examination

The clinical examination includes a general physical examination to rule out other injuries, for which medical consultation should be sought, and a comprehensive regional examination of the head and neck.

Neurologic assessment of level of consciousness, orientation to time and place, and presence of intraoral and extraoral paresthesia is critical. Visual field integrity, including the reaction of pupils to light and accommodation, is evaluated. Palpation of the facial skeleton provides opportunity to describe bony asymmetry, crepitus, mobility, depression or tenderness over the mandible, maxilla, malar bones, and zygomatic arches. The range of motion of the mandible is described. The condyles are palpated during excursions. Positive findings suggestive of a facial fracture require further investigation, and a maxillofacial surgical consultation may be indicated.

All intraoral and extraoral soft tissue wounds are recorded, with special attention to the implantation of foreign matter. Extraoral and peripheral intraoral soft tissue wounds are dressed and reduced if they are not within the field of the dentoalveolar injury; if a component of the dental trauma, they are treated subsequent to initial dentoalveolar immobilization. Closure of soft tissue wounds in close proximity (e.g., lip lacerations) usually is done after the dentoalveolar injuries are stabilized, to prevent undue stress on the suture lines resulting in a poor surgical outcome. Follow the rule for repair of wounds: hard tissues first, then soft tissues.

The occlusion is evaluated carefully for any suggestion of jaw fracture or dental prematurities as a result of tooth displacement. The teeth are examined for crown crazing, fractures, and pulp exposures. Displacement of all teeth is recorded and direction of dental displacement described. Horizontal and vertical tooth mobility is evaluated and recorded. Positive reaction to percussion and palpation as well as all positive and notable negative findings are documented.

1. **Regional examination of head and neck**
   a. **Neuromuscular examination:** The patient should be alert and oriented to time and place, pupils should be equally round and reactive to light and accommodation (PERRLA), extraocular muscles should be intact (EOMI). Examine for presence of obvious ocular lesions; review integrity of visual fields and record diplopia or blurred vision; grossly examine cranial nerves 1 through 12 for intactness without paresthesia; and evaluate muscles of facial expression.

b. **Examination of skin of face and neck:** Examine for normal facial pigmentation and texture without swelling, masses, lesions, lacerations, or inflammatory processes.

c. **Examination of facial bones:** Examine for bony symmetry, crepitus, mobility, and depression or tenderness over the mandible, maxilla, or zygomaticomaxillary complex. Describe mandibular envelope of motion and palpability of condyles.

d. **Adenopathy:** Describe palpable lymph nodes: location, size, tenderness, and mobility.

e. **Soft tissue examination:** Evaluate the lips, buccal mucosa, vestibules, palate, and floor of mouth. Describe color, contour, masses and lesions.

f. **Examination of the tongue:** Describe size, color, papillation, and texture, and presence of masses, lesions, lacerations, or deviations from normal function.

g. **Examination of salivary glands:** Evaluate the parotid, submandibular, and sublingual glands. Size, shape, and texture should be normal, without any palpable masses. Ducts should be patent, with copious flow of clear saliva.

h. **Gingival examination:** Describe color, contour, and texture, and presence of masses, lesions, lacerations, or bleeding.

i. **Examination of teeth and occlusion:** Describe existing occlusion and any discrepancies. Chart existing dentition and any dental disorders, including fractured, displaced, and missing teeth.

2. **Summary of clinical examination of dentoalveolar injuries**

a. **Palpate the facial skeleton** and record extraoral wounds. Palpate the maxilla, mandible, zygomaticomaxillary complex and record abnormalities in occlusion. Evaluate the mandibular envelope of motion.

b. **Record intraoral soft tissue injuries** and rule out presence of foreign material in the lips and cheeks.

    c. **Examine tooth crowns** for crazing, fractures, pulp exposures, and discoloration.

    d. **Note any tooth displacement** and evaluate. Record horizontal and vertical tooth mobility.

    e. **Record reaction to percussion and palpation** of teeth.

C. **Radiographic examination**

Radiographic examination of dentoalveolar trauma is essential for the detection of skeletal or alveolar fractures and of tooth fragments or other foreign bodies within soft tissues. Undetected root fractures are often visualized, and the proximity of the pulp tissue to enamel and dentinal injuries can be determined. The degree of tooth displacement can be visualized. Clinically diagnosed facial fractures require maxillofacial surgical consultation along with skull films and maxillary or mandibular series as indicated. Panoramic radiographs are exceptionally valuable to evaluate trauma to the mandible, maxilla, and dentoalveolar complex.

Diagnostic radiographic evaluation of dental trauma has traditionally been achieved by periapical or occlusal views of the affected areas. Multiple views, using a variety of angulations, are an excellent source of diagnostic information. If intraoral films are not easily obtainable, extraoral views are taken, including inferior oblique and lateral (sagittal) projections. For a sagittal exposure, the central beam should be aligned perpendicular to the structure in question and exposure time increased by 50%. The film can be taped to the patient's face to facilitate stabilization. Soft tissue radiographs can help rule out the presence of foreign bodies or tooth fragments within those tissues. Generally, decreasing exposure times by 30% to 50% provides adequate soft tissue contrast.

II. **DENTOALVEOLAR INJURY TO PRIMARY DENTITION**

Traumatic injuries to the primary dentition provoke a great deal of anxiety on the part of parents because of the young age of the child and the presence of copious bleeding, even with minor soft tissue wounds. Reassuring and calming the parents will facilitate obtaining an accurate and contributory dental and medical history. Clinical examination is often difficult. If the child is younger than 4 years of age, being held in the parent's lap often provides needed physical and emotional support and assists in mildly restraining the child during clinical inspection. Inability to obtain a history from the child and lack of accurate response to diagnostic measures will make the diagnosis of primary tooth trauma more difficult.

A. Concussive and subluxation injuries

   1. Diagnosis: The diagnosis of **concussive tooth trauma** is difficult and is based on history or visualization of a dental impact injury. Often the episode is unobserved and is not recognized for an extended period until tooth discoloration, a potential sequela, prompts consultation. Acute diagnosis is based on marked sensitivity of the tooth to percussion or manipulation and lack of mobility or displacement. The radiographic examination is unremarkable. In young children, reliable elicitation of positive percussion sensitivity can be problematic.

      Subluxation injuries are easily diagnosed. The tooth is abnormally mobile in the horizontal plane but is not displaced. Gingival cuff bleeding is a common parental chief complaint, and indicates damage to the periodontium. A maxillary radiograph may demonstrate an increase in the width of the periodontal ligament space.

   2. Treatment: The initial maxillary occlusal radiograph is used as a baseline for future evaluation. The child is placed on a soft diet for 1 week to decrease percussion sensitivity and prevent further insult. No stabilization is required.

   3. Complications: Concussion and subluxation injuries often result in pulpal hemorrhage and subsequent coronal discoloration, the result of hemoglobin breakdown products entering the dentinal tubules. Initially the crown has a pinkish hue, which generally changes to gray-blue over time. Coronal discoloration alone is not indicative of necrotic pulp in the primary dentition; however, a large percentage of teeth that sustain a deep gray discoloration become necrotic. Some teeth develop a yellow opaque tint if the pulp chamber and canal become obliterated, due to stimulation of secondary dentin formation; more than 70% of such teeth remain vital.

The patient is seen 1 to 2 weeks after the initial injury for evaluation of coronal discoloration or perceived symptoms. If any coronal discoloration occurs, the patient should return for evaluation immediately. At 3 months a second maxillary occlusal radiograph is obtained and compared with that taken at initial presentation. Potential changes may include internal or external root resorption or periapical rarefaction. Clinical signs of pulpal degeneration include pain and discomfort, increased tooth mobility, and gingival or periapical swelling and draining fistulas.

Discolored primary teeth should undergo pulp therapy when there are radiographic or clinical signs of pulpal necrosis. Pulp therapy consists of a complete pulpectomy, with copious irrigation and placement of a formocresol pellet or paper point for 5 minutes, followed by complete obturation with a resorbable zinc oxide and eugenol paste. If purulent drainage is present, antibiotic therapy should be considered. Due to the prognosis of this procedure, and a predicted success rate of only 50%, extraction may be considered for teeth with excessive mobility or significant external or internal root resorption.

It is difficult to predict the potential sequelae in teeth sustaining concussion and subluxation injuries. Pulpal degeneration with positive radiographic or clinical findings may occur immediately following the injury or not for many years. The patient is followed up every 3 to 6 months, with periodic radiographic evaluation. Parents are instructed to observe for crown discoloration, increasing tooth mobility, or development of a fistula associated with the injured tooth. Although acute periapical abscess may result in discomfort, posttraumatic sequelae to the primary dentition often are asymptomatic and may delay presentation. The insidious nature of these injuries may not be appreciated or recognized. After an initial complaint of tooth discoloration a retrospective diagnosis of concussion or subluxation injury may be made. Once identified, monitoring and follow-up care are consistent with that for an original injury. An attempt is made to determine the predisposing episode that resulted in the development of sequelae, to establish a time frame for baseline comparison.

B. Crown fracture

Severity of crown fractures ranges from mild enamel crazing to extensive involvement of the dental pulp. The Ellis classification of coronal fractures is used to grade this type of dental injury. This classification system describes the extent of coronal fracture by the presence of enamel, dentin, or pulp involvement. Crown fractures in the primary dentition are not common and generally are superficial, involving only enamel or a minimal amount of dentin. This is a result of the compliance of the dental alveolus in the child and the tendency of traumatic forces to be distributed from the tooth to the alveolar bone, generally resulting in tooth luxation rather than crown fracture.

1. **Diagnosis:** The diagnosis of coronal fractures is predicated on clinical inspection. A descriptive narrative and schematic drawing defining the extent of the injury and its proximity to the dental pulp is recommended. The tooth is examined for mobility, which is suggestive of possible root fracture or alveolar bone injury.

2. **Treatment:** Treatment includes preoperative radiographs to rule out concomitant injuries and for baseline documentation. Crown crazing does not require immediate therapy. Minor enamel fractures can be treated with enamelplasty. Fractures involving a significant amount of enamel loss or extending into the dentin without involving the pulp require sedative dressing and restorative treatment. A calcium hydroxide base is applied to exposed dentin and maintained with a glass ionomer liner or an acid-

etched bonded resin. If possible, a full composite restoration can be placed to maintain the sedative dressing and restore the tooth to normal contour. When pulpal involvement is detected, a classic 5-minute formocresol pulpotomy or pulpectomy must be performed. Following obturation and temporization with zinc oxide and eugenol paste, the tooth can be restored to normal contour.

3. **Complications:** Ellis class I and II coronal fractures are observed closely for development of pulpal necrosis. A 3-month follow-up including a periapical radiograph is essential, followed by reevaluation every 6 months. If pulp necrosis is noted any time after the injury, a pulpectomy with zinc oxide and eugenol obturation is necessary. Teeth receiving classic formocresol pulpotomy or pulpectomy at the time of the initial injury require annual clinical and radiographic follow-up examination, and generally the prognosis is good.

C. **Root fracture**

Root fractures in the primary dentition rarely occur and are problematic. The prognosis for maintaining the tooth depends on the location of the fracture and the treatment method selected.

1. **Diagnosis:** Root fractures may be suspected when excessive coronal mobility is present. Definitive diagnosis is made via periapical or occlusal radiography. A single film may be inadequate, and a lateral or sagittal film may prove valuable. Discontinuity of the periodontal ligament and linear or circular radiolucent lines crossing the root surface are important radiographic diagnostic markers.

2. **Treatment:** Teeth with minimally mobile coronal segments can be maintained without immediate therapy. The patient is placed on a soft diet for several weeks, and a regular reevaluation schedule is maintained. Teeth with moderate or excessive mobility should be extracted. If the apical segment can easily be visualized and removed without damage to the developing permanent tooth bud, an attempt is made to retrieve it. When extraction of the root fragment

may prove difficult, the apical fragment may be left in place and observed periodically for normal resorption.

3. **Complications:** Root fracture in the primary dentition carries a poor prognosis. Teeth with minimal coronal mobility often devitalize and extraction is required. When an apical fragment remains within the alveolus, regular clinical and radiographic follow-up is necessary. Any evidence of infection or abscess formation requires immediate intervention. Apical root fragments generally resorb naturally or spontaneously exfoliate without complication.

D. **Dental luxation**

Luxation injuries to the primary dentition are common, accounting for more than 60% of all pediatric dentoalveolar injuries. The thinness of the alveolar bone facilitates absorption of kinetic energy, thus cushioning the tooth itself. The critical factors appear to be the force and direction of impact. The most frequent luxation injury is intrusion of maxillary primary teeth in infants and preschool children.

1. **Diagnosis:** Determining the kind of luxation injury is vital, because prognosis and treatment are specific to the varying types. The diagnosis is made on clinical assessment and location of the displaced teeth. Location of the apex of the traumatized primary tooth and its proximity to the developing permanent tooth bud is critical. Accurate diagnosis is invalid without positive and definitive identification of the resting position of the tooth apex. Often the resting position of the crown will translate to root location. Intraoral radiographs and lateral films are critical in identifying the anteroposterior apical relationship of the primary tooth to the cortical plates and developing permanent teeth. Sagittal exposures are essential, because it is impossible to visualize this relationship with periapical and occlusal films. Periapical or maxillary occlusal films should be obtained to establish a baseline for future periodontal comparison and early recognition of external root resorption.

2. **Treatment:** Maxillary anterior intrusive luxation is the most frequently seen primary tooth luxation injury. Intrusive injuries resulting in close proximity of the primary tooth apex to a developing permanent tooth require immediate extraction. Severely intruded maxillary primary incisors with minor to moderate buccal plate perforation may be observed. Fully impacted primary teeth that severely perforate the cortical plate and lie solely within soft tissue of the mucobuccal fold should be extracted. Labial, lingual, and laterally luxated primary teeth should be repositioned as soon as possible. Because of the compliance of alveolar bone in pediatric patients, this is easily accomplished by grasping the alveolar bone between finger and thumb and briskly snapping it back into proper arch relationship. If traumatic occlusion persists and reduction is impossible, the tooth must be extracted. Stabilization of luxated primary teeth is generally not necessary following reduction. If excessive mobility remains after a reduction attempt, extraction is recommended.

3. **Complications:** Intrusive luxation of primary teeth that meets the acute care criteria for maintenance generally re-erupts within 2 to 3 weeks after the injury. Once acceptably repositioned, these teeth are closely observed for development of pulpal necrosis. If re-eruption does not occur within a reasonable period of time, surgical extraction must be considered.

   Laterally, labially, and lingually luxated teeth that have been successfully repositioned are followed up closely. Decreasing mobility should occur after the first few weeks. If excessive mobility persists, the tooth should be removed. Radiographs are taken 3 months after trauma, then at 6 and 12 months. A high likelihood of pulpal necrosis exists within the first few months. Radiographic or clinical signs of pulpal necrosis or external root resorption may occur later. Any luxated tooth that develops clinical or radiographic signs of pulp necrosis or periodontal ligament breakdown requires immediate endodontic therapy or extraction.

E. Avulsion

1. **Diagnosis:** The diagnosis of complete exarticulation of a tooth is made by clinical inspection of the affected tooth or via a radiograph of the voided alveolar socket. Occasionally apical root fragments remain, and their presence should be verified.

2. **Treatment:** Primary teeth that are avulsed should not be replanted. Hemostasis should be established. Any remaining root or tooth fragments are removed, if easily and atraumatically accomplished, or they can be left and observed for normal resorption or exfoliation. The missing tooth should be located.

3. **Complications:** The prognosis for replanted primary teeth is extremely poor, often resulting in multiple complications (e.g., ankylosis) that inhibit or deflect eruption of succedaneous teeth. *Teeth that have been replanted should be immediately extracted.* Esthetic and space maintenance considerations can be made depending on the age of the child and the location of the avulsion.

III. DENTOALVEOLAR INJURY TO PERMANENT DENTITION

Trauma to the permanent dentition has lifelong implications, and appropriate acute care management has direct impact on prognosis. Timely follow-up care and close observation, particularly during the first year, affects prognosis and the potential maintenance of the traumatized tooth.

Often dentoalveolar trauma to the permanent dentition is associated with significant craniofacial or systemic injury. A thorough physical assessment and regional examination of the head and neck are performed. Positive neurologic or systemic physical findings warrant immediate medical consultation. Once the patient is stable, management of the dentoalveolar injury can be addressed. An avulsed tooth should be replanted while consultation is sought.

Splinting and stabilization of luxated and avulsed permanent teeth play a critical part in management and prognosis. Currently recommended splinting techniques include acid-etched composite resins with or without orthodontic wires and brackets, nylon line splints, and elaborate basket suturing. Criteria for selecting a splint to reduce dental luxations and avulsions include ease of applicability and removal, flexibility to allow for normal physiologic tooth movement, and cleansability. Rigid splinting often results in nonfunctional periodontal ligament fibers that are parallel to the length of the tooth and predispose to the development of ankylosis.

Calcium hydroxide interim obturation often is required following pulp extirpation and pulpectomy. USP grade calcium hydroxide should be mixed with either sterile water or local anesthetic solution and 20% barium sulfate or zinc oxide to increase radiopacity. Prepackaged commercial preparations in syringe form facilitate ease of placement. Calcium hydroxide base or linear materials should not be used for canal obturation, because of bioavailability concerns and difficulty in removing hard-setting materials.

1. **Criteria for splint selection** for dental luxations and avulsions include the following:
   a. **Placement:** Ease and rapidity of splint insertion and removal are essential.
   b. **Stabilization:** The splint should be nonrigid to allow for physiologic tooth movement and prevention of ankylosis. Only passive forces should be placed on the injured teeth.
   c. **Cleansability:** To prevent further gingival and periodontal inflammation, the splint should be supragingival. This allows for normal home care to promote plaque control and healing of the periodontium.
   d. **Accessibility:** The splint should allow endodontic access and visibility.
   e. **Maintenance:** Stabilization periods are based on the injury sustained; however, the shortest time frame necessary is most preferable and efficacious. Splints should be removed as soon as the tooth is stable enough to be maintained without assistance.

2. **Splints recommended** for treatment of dental luxations and avulsions include:
   a. **Composite resin splints:**
      (1) Acid-etched design.
      (2) With or without orthodontic brackets or
          wires.
   b. **Nylon line splints:**
      (1) Monofilament 50 lb test line.
      (2) Held in place with bonded composite resin
          on labial tooth surface.
      (3) Highly flexible; permit function of the sup-
          porting periodontium.
   c. **Suture splints:**
      (1) Excellent for acute care management and
          unmanageable children.
   d. **Removable appliances** with incisal stabilizing
      wires:
      (1) For placement subsequent to initial reduc-
          tion.
      (2) In cases where acute stabilization is difficult
          or when a nonrecommended splint was used.
A. **Concussion and subluxation injuries**
   1. **Diagnosis:** Concussion and subluxation injuries to
   the permanent dentition are common. The diagnosis
   is made on documented history of traumatic impact
   to the teeth without evidence of displacement or
   altered occlusion. Concussion injuries show no discernible mobility. Subluxated teeth exhibit detectable mobility without evidence of tooth displacement. Radiographs of subluxated teeth often demonstrate widening of the periodontal ligament space,
   whereas teeth that have sustained a concussion injury are radiographically unremarkable.
   2. **Treatment:** Acute care management includes an
   adequate radiographic survey of the affected teeth
   for baseline purposes, and soft dietary intake for at
   least 1 week or until percussion sensitivity abates.
   Splinting of teeth is not necessary, and in fact is
   contraindicated. The patient is reminded to maintain
   impeccable oral hygiene to prevent retrograde bacte-

rial invasion through the gingival sulcus into the periodontal ligament space.

3. **Complications:** Close follow-up is essential to detect early signs of pulpal necrosis and devitalization. Immature teeth with "blunderbuss" apices have a better pulpal prognosis than teeth with complete apical closure. After a concussion or subluxation injury the patient is followed up closely for the first 2 weeks. Six weeks after the injury vitality testing is generally diagnostic and reliable, and should be performed. If pulp testing indicates devitalization the pulp is accessed and a calcium hydroxide pulpectomy performed. Interim calcium hydroxide pulpectomies are generally recommended for 6 to 12 months before final obturation is considered.

Pulp testing is often problematic, particularly in children, and requires a variety of approaches, including electronic pulp testing, application of hot and cold substances, and definitively by initiating a test cavity without local anesthesia prior to initiation of endodontic therapy. In teeth that test vital, periodic radiographic observation is necessary and performed at 3, 6, and 12 months. Internal or external root resorption is indicative of pulpal necrosis or significant damage to the supporting periodontal apparatus. After 1 year, continued semiannual follow-up is essential. Severe internal or external root replacement-resorption may occur without detectable clinical signs and symptoms at any time after the injury. Clinical follow up schedules must be adhered to for positive results. Occasionally the injury produces stimulation of reparative dentin and resultant pulpal obliteration. Since a percentage of these teeth devitalize and are difficult to treat by conventional endodontic measures, early detection and pulp extirpation are desirable. If pulpal obliteration occurs and the tooth becomes symptomatic, an apical surgical procedure may be necessary.

B. Crown fracture

Crown fractures in the permanent dentition are common, and are graded using the Ellis classification. Treatment may be complicated by pulpal involvement. Prognosis and treatment of pulpally involved teeth with immature root development vary significantly from that in teeth with adequate secondary dentin but incomplete apical closure. The stage of tooth development must be closely evaluated.

1. **Diagnosis:** Diagnosis and classification of coronal fractures require careful clinical inspection. Detection of minute pulpal involvement by tactile examination is critical. Radiographs are essential to rule out concomitant root or alveolar fractures.

2. **Treatment:** Initial treatment is dictated by the presence or absence of pulpal involvement.

   a. **Fractures limited to enamel and dentin:** In Ellis class I or class II fractures in which the pulp chamber has not been violated, treatment consists of restoring the tooth to normal contour and function. Calcium hydroxide should be placed on all exposed dentinal surfaces. Glass ionomer liners can be considered for placement on exposed dentin remote from pulpal proximity to improve retention of the base and final restoration. Generally, acid-etched bonded composite restorations can be placed at the time of injury to provide an immediate esthetic result that will greatly reduce patient and family anxiety.

      A broken off tooth segment can be reattached using acid-etched resin. No beveling of either tooth surface is necessary, and the broken segment is luted in place with a bonding agent after enamel preparation. Final retention is good, and esthetic results are often quite remarkable.

      In cases where retention and esthetics are deemed adequate, composite angle fracture repairs have long-term implications. When a significant amount of tooth structure is absent or esthetic results are problematic, porcelain veneers or full crown coverage may be considered.

b. **Coronal fractures with pulpal involvement:**
   When crown fracture results in pulp exposure,
   multiple treatment options are available, depending on the extent of pulpal injury, stage of root
   development, and age of the patient.

c. **Immature teeth with incomplete apicogenesis:**
   Teeth with open apices and an inadequate zone
   of primary and secondary dentin produce a restorative dilemma if devitalization occurs. With
   inadequate dentin formation the tooth resembles
   an unsupported tube of cementum and dentin and
   is extremely fragile and unable to accommodate
   a post and core for future restorative needs.
   Therefore treatment is directed at encouraging
   normal secondary dentin formation and apicogenesis.

   Pulp exposure in teeth with minimal dentin
   formation and wide open apices are treated by
   calcium hydroxide pulpotomy or partial pulpotomy at the time of the injury. Partial pulpotomy
   is performed by removing pulpal tissue 2 mm
   below the site of exposure or until fresh bleeding
   is noted, as in cases where there is delay in presentation. Pulp is extirpated with high-speed rotary diamond burs. Hemostasis is established
   with sterile cotton pledget pressure. **Local anesthetic agents are not injected into the pulp.**
   Once hemostasis is established using local pressure, calcium hydroxide should be placed directly against the exposed vital pulpal tissue and
   sealed with zinc oxide and eugenol paste. Frequent radiographic follow-up is performed, with
   close scrutiny for evidence of internal root resorption. Success is determined by a radiographically discernible calcific border between the sedative dressing and pulp chamber. It is not necessary to reapply the calcium hydroxide or to clinically assess the presence of the calcific border.
   This treatment can be considered definitive.

   In immature teeth with adequate primary and
   secondary dentin formation and incomplete api-

cal closure, treatment is directed at apicogenesis, because the root is well formed and of adequate thickness for restorative needs. Although calcium hydroxide pulpotomy may be performed in these cases, the classic Frank technique, that is, placement of calcium hydroxide to the measured apex of the tooth, to obtain apical closure prior to final endodontic obturation may be selected. Pulpectomy at least 2 mm short of the apex is performed, and calcium hydroxide is placed by syringe to the measured apex of the tooth. These teeth are evaluated radiographically at 2, 6, and 12 weeks for determination of continued apical closure. Periodic replacement of calcium hydroxide is highly recommended. Success is based on continuation of apical closure without evidence of progressive external root resorption or periapical disease.

d. **Mature teeth with complete apicogenesis:** Teeth with fully formed roots with closed apices demonstrating traumatic pulpal involvement are assessed for extent of pulp exposure. Limited pulp exposure can be treated initially with direct calcium hydroxide pulp caps within 24 hours of the injury. Teeth with significant pulpal exposure should be endodontically treated in conventional fashion. Conventional endodontic treatment for teeth with minute pulp exposure is an acceptable alternative to pulp capping.

3. **Complications:** Calcium hydroxide direct pulp capping and pulpotomy in young permanent teeth are radiographically and clinically successful in a large majority of cases. The success of direct pulp capping in mature teeth with closed apices is critically compared with the predictable success rate of conventional endodontic therapy. With careful follow-up, complications of direct pulp capping can be intercepted and reversed with standard endodontic approaches. In young permanent teeth with incomplete root formation exhibiting limited pulp exposure, partial or complete calcium hydroxide pulpot-

omy has been successful. Formation of calcific dentinal bridges without evidence of clinical or radiographic signs of internal or external root resorption may be considered clinically successful. These barriers do not require clinical inspection. Complete hard tissue barriers are protective and generally exhibit no evidence of pulpitis even in the presence of histologic dead tracts. Pulpotomy and direct pulp capping should not be considered as interim treatment in the absence of clinical or radiographic signs of failure, and therefore may obviate the need for conventional root canal therapy.

C. Root fracture

Root fractures in the permanent dentition represent less than 10% of all dentoalveolar injuries affecting the permanent teeth. They are common in patients aged 11 to 20 years, but are rarely seen in younger persons because the elasticity of the alveolar socket predisposes these teeth to luxation injuries. In general, maintenance of pulp vitality in teeth with root fractures is not unexpected, as opposed to teeth that have been luxated or avulsed.

Root fractures are most often seen in the apical or middle third of the root, and rarely in the coronal third. Root fractures in the coronal third carry the poorest prognosis because of the likelihood of communication of the fracture site with the gingival sulcus. Teeth with fractured roots often undergo partial or complete pulp canal obliteration without development of pulpal necrosis.

1. **Diagnosis:** Permanent teeth with root fractures often appear mildly extruded from the alveolar socket, or the crown may exhibit slight lingual displacement. The tooth may be mobile, depending on the location of the fracture.

    Radiographic examination is critical to diagnosis. Anterior occlusal projections are generally most productive. Multiple angulations are recommended, and depending on the oblique nature of the fracture site, will generally project as a single radiolucent line. Occasionally a diffuse circular or ellipsoid radiolucency may be noted as a result of the angle of the central X-ray beam projecting obliquely to the fracture site. Occasionally root fractures may not be immediately evident but are noted on subsequent radiographic surveys. This is probably due to extravasation of blood into or the development of granulation tissue at the fracture site, resulting in displacement of the coronal segment. Root fractures are often associated with alveolar bone injuries, especially in the mandibular anterior region, and detection of concomitant dentoalveolar injuries will affect the treatment course. Coronal root fractures have a poor prognosis.

2. **Treatment:** In contrast to dental luxations and avulsions, the objective of therapy of root fractures is rigid immobilization for 2 to 3 months. Initial treatment is directed at reduction of displaced fragments and rigid stabilization. Digital manipulation and reduction immediately after the injury are necessary and usually easily accomplished. If resistance is felt, a concomitant alveolar fracture is probably present, and manipulation of the fractured socket should be attempted. Once reduction is performed, radiographic confirmation is recommended.

   Rigid fixation is best accomplished using acid-etched bonded composite materials in bulk with or without heavy orthodontic wires and brackets. These should be strong and nonflexible to allow for hard tissue consolidation at the fracture site. Throughout the rigid stabilization phase the teeth are observed radiographically and frequent vitality testing is performed to detect the development of pulpal necrosis. A negative vitality response immediately after injury is expected. A slow return to a normal vital response can generally be anticipated. The patient is placed on a soft diet for a minimum of 1 to 2 weeks and is advised to avoid any significant incisal forces throughout the stabilization period.

3. **Complications:** Teeth with root fractures may develop signs or symptoms of pulpal necrosis or external root resorption at the site of the fracture. Pain,

percussion sensitivity, and radiographic evidence of increasing separation of the fractured segments or external root resorption at the fracture site are poor prognostic indicators and are usually evident within 2 to 3 months. A majority of teeth with simple root fractures maintain pulpal vitality.

Factors that contribute to pulpal necrosis include extensive extrusion of the coronal segment, nonrigid splinting, and fracture of the coronal third in communication with the gingival sulcus. The prevalence of pulpal vitality may be due to revascularization of the pulp from the periodontal ligament at the fracture site and the ability of the site to accommodate pulpal edema. A majority of these teeth may undergo partial or complete pulpal obliteration over time, and as early as 9 to 12 months after injury. Pulpal obliteration is generally completed within 1 to 2 years. Clinically the crown has an opaque yellowish hue. Generally these teeth maintain vitality, and secondary pulpal necrosis is rare. If symptoms develop, a surgical apical procedure may be necessary.

Rigid immobilization allows for the development of a uniting callous made up of dentin, osteodentin, or cementum. Most often this hard tissue incompletely bridges the defect. Interspersed throughout the bridge is connective tissue originating from the periodontal ligament. Therefore, even in successful cases, complete union of the root surfaces is never achieved, although full continuity of the periodontal ligament space may be seen surrounding the hard tissue and connective tissue matrix.

Pulpal degeneration occurs in a minority of teeth with root fractures, and is generally limited to the coronal segment, with vital apical pulp tissue remaining. Pulp extirpation of the coronal segment is performed and obturated with calcium hydroxide for 12 months. Once clinical and radiographic signs of healing occur and there is no longer evidence of continued external root resorption and associated alveolar bone radiolucencies, final obturation can be attempted.

If a hard tissue callous at the fracture site does not develop, along with radiographic or clinical signs of disunion or abscess formation, obturation of the coronal segment with root amputation is recommended. If the fracture is in the coronal third of the root, consideration should be given to amputating the crown to the fracture site, performing conventional endodontic therapy on the apical segment, and orthodontically extruding the obturated segment prior to placement of a final restoration. If the prognosis in any of these contingencies is poor, extraction and prosthetic replacement may be indicated.

D. Luxation

Luxation injuries are common, accounting for as many as 40% of all dentoalveolar injuries to the permanent dentition. Luxated mature permanent teeth have an extremely high potential for development of pulpal necrosis. Secondary pulp necrosis in luxated teeth that have undergone pulpal obliteration is common.

Any injury resulting in displacement of the teeth will cause damage or fracture to the adjacent alveolar bone. This is often problematic, because the treatment of true segmental alveolar fractures varies significantly from that for luxated injuries. The major difference relates to the site of the fracture. In luxated injuries the alveolar socket and supporting periodontal structures are severely compromised, and treatment is directed toward reestablishment of the normal relationship of the tooth to the periodontium and supporting alveolus. In a true alveolar fracture the objective is to achieve bone-to-bone union. In both types of injuries, coexistence and overlap of either diagnosis is likely and the clinician must direct attention to the primary problem.

1. **Diagnosis:** Diagnosis of luxated injuries is based on thorough clinical examination and radiographic assessment. The direction and degree of luxation are critical because treatment and prognosis are predicated on these findings.

Luxations are generally classified as intrusive;

extrusive, or partially avulsed; and lateral, with documentation of the posttraumatic anatomic resting position.

a. **Intrusive luxations** can be diagnosed by observing for discrepancies in the incisal or occlusal relationship of adjacent teeth. This diagnosis is easily confirmed radiographically, because the periodontal ligament space is often obliterated. Teeth may not exhibit any mobility due to the impaction, and percussion response has been described as "metallic." If a permanent central incisor is intruded, inspection of the floor of the nose should be done to identify any bleeding and the possibility of protrusion of the apex of the tooth into the nasal cavity.

b. **Extrusive luxations** are essentially partial avulsions. Clinically they are generally very mobile, with an obvious discrepancy in the occlusal plane. Radiographically, the apical portion of the tooth appears displaced from the alveolar socket and a general increase in the width of periodontal ligament space may be evident.

c. **In lateral luxations** the resting position of the root and apex should be determined. This can be done by reviewing the resting crown position and extrapolating the root position or by multiple radiographic exposures including lateral (sagittal) films. By the very nature of the injury, concomitant alveolar bone fracture must be anticipated.

2. **Treatment:** Intrusive luxations have the poorest prognosis, because of extensive injury to the root apex and floor of the alveolar socket. Expeditious acute care is essential. Intruded permanent teeth do not have the potential to spontaneously re-erupt unless they are extremely immature with wide open apices.

Because of the injuries sustained, pulpal necrosis can be anticipated in all cases with fully formed apices. Treatment should be directed toward endodontic therapy. Often surgical exposure is necessary because the tooth is not easily visualized. Sometimes orthodontically induced re-eruption may be necessary to access the pulp chamber. Complete pulpectomy with debridement and copious irrigation is performed 24 to 48 hours after the injury. Calcium hydroxide obturation should be deferred until 7 to 10 days after the injury. Immediate orthodontic consideration must be given to mechanical repositioning of intruded teeth with closed apices. Failure to initiate extrusive mechanics will result in ankylosis. Expedience is the rule. Extrusive and lateral luxations are immediately reduced and repositioned and a nonrigid splint placed to maintain their normal occlusal and physiologic relationships. Teeth that are mildly laterally displaced or have wide open apices can be observed for signs of pulpal necrosis. Extrusively and laterally luxated teeth with moderate to severe displacement can be treated endodontically 24 to 48 hours after reduction and stabilization. After pulpal extirpation the canal is carefully debrided and copiously irrigated, and left without medications for 7 to 10 days, when obturation of the canal to the measured apex with calcium hydroxide is performed.

3. **Complications:** Intrusive luxations are the most difficult to manage and have the poorest prognosis. Damage to the apical region of the tooth often results in the stimulation of progressive external replacement-resorption, a phenomenon often leading to ankylosis. Ankylosis also develops in cases where orthodontic mechanical extrusion is unduly delayed, and further attempts to orthodontically reposition the tooth are generally unsuccessful.

   Immature teeth with wide open apices have some eruptive potential. If no eruption is noted within the first 4 weeks, orthodontic therapy should be initiated. These teeth are followed up very closely for radiographic or clinical signs of pulpal degeneration or necrosis and are promptly treated with pulpectomy and calcium hydroxide obturation. Mature teeth with closed apices that have been pulpectomized, obturated with calcium hydroxide, and orthodontically treated are clinically and radiographically observed during the first year of treatment. Orthodontic forced eruption is easily accomplished and can be completed with 6 to 8 weeks of mechanical therapy. Within the first year of treatment calcium hydroxide should be replaced after 3 weeks, then bimonthly, or more frequently if it is apparent that the tooth is no longer adequately obturated. Conventional endodontic obturation can be considered after 1 year if the tooth is clinically asymptomatic and free of radiographic apical disease or after cessation of external root resorption. Teeth that have sustained extrusive or lateral luxation injuries requiring stabilization splints should be considered for splint removal no longer than 2 weeks after the injury, and sooner if the injured teeth remain firm without assistance. It has been shown that shorter stabilization periods are preferable and result in fewer cases of irreversible root replacement-resorption.

Immature teeth or mildly luxated mature teeth in which immediate endodontic therapy is deferred require close observation. Radiographs of these teeth are taken at 2, 6, and 12 weeks, then every 6 months for the first few years.

Pulp testing should be initiated 6 weeks after the injury, then periodically performed. Evidence of pulp devitalization requires pulpal extirpation and a 1-year course of calcium hydroxide obturation.

In all endodontically treated luxated and extruded teeth, final obturation should be deferred for the first year. Calcium hydroxide can be replaced 3 weeks after initial placement, then bimonthly. After 1 year, final obturation can be considered if no signs of external root replacement-resorption or other periapical disease is evident.

E. Avulsion

No other situation in dental practice is more emergent or requires more prompt and well-directed treatment than avulsion of a permanent tooth. There is a direct relationship between the extra-alveolar duration and replantation, and survival of avulsed teeth. The prognosis is guarded to favorable in teeth replanted within the first 60 minutes, guarded to fair in teeth exarticulated for more than 60 minutes, and extremely poor in those avulsed longer than 2 hours.

Factors that influence prognosis include delay in replantation, improper handling of the avulsed tooth, method of stabilization, and timing and selection of endodontic therapy. Comminution and fractures of the alveolar socket also impact negatively on successful outcome, as may the storage medium used during the extra-alveolar phase. Avulsions account for 0.5% to 16% of all dentoalveolar injuries to the permanent dentition. Exarticulation occurs predominantly in children between 7 and 10 years of age, and most often involves the maxillary incisors. Erupting teeth are most susceptible to avulsion because of immaturity of supporting periodontal ligaments.

1. **Diagnosis:** In establishing the diagnosis, it is critical to know the patient's age and whether it is a permanent or primary tooth that is avulsed. Primary teeth should not be replanted. If the patient presents directly, cursory clinical examination including inspection of the avulsed tooth is definitive. Pretreatment radiographs are contraindicated because they consume precious extra-alveolar time. It is extremely important that the extra-alveolar duration be noted and documented.

2. **Treatment**
   a. **Telephone consultation:** If you are contacted by phone, clear and specific instructions must be given. Prompt reinsertion is paramount. The tooth is irrigated without manipulating the root surface. The best irrigation solution in a non-office setting is the patient's saliva; however, milk or saline solution may be suggested as an alternative. **Tap water is detrimental to the periodontal ligament.** If no irrigation solutions are available, reinsertion without irrigation is preferable to prolonging the extra-alveolar period.

   If the patient cannot manage or tolerate reinsertion, a transport medium is essential. Placement of the tooth in the patient's buccal vestibule is the best alternative, followed by placement of the tooth in the vestibule of the person accompanying the patient; if both alternatives are unacceptable, the tooth should be placed in saline solution or milk. The patient is instructed to come to the dental office immediately. If replantation was achieved, the patient is instructed to keep the tooth in place with finger or gauze pressure.

b. Office consultation: When the patient presents directly to the office, expeditious replantation is performed. The tooth is carefully irrigated with sterile physiologic saline solution, and an attempt must be made to avoid contact or manipulation of the root surface. If the tooth meets resistance on reinsertion, check for comminution of the alveolar socket. Manipulation of the socket using digital pressure may be necessary to permit replantation. Local anesthesia is usually not necessary but may be administered in selected cases. A postinsertion radiograph is taken. Following replantation, a nonrigid splint should be applied and an effort made to passively maintain tooth position.

Adequate stability after reinsertion is not unusual. In uncooperative children it may be sufficient to maintain the tooth with a simple sling suture over the incisal edge. If the extra-alveolar duration is more than 2 hours the tooth should be irrigated with sterile saline solution and placed in 2.55% neutral sodium fluoride solution for 20 minutes before replantation.

Tetanus immunization history is closely reviewed, and a booster dose administered if necessary (see Table 3–1). Antibiotic therapy with penicillin for 1 week is recommended because of contamination inherent to the injury.

3. Complications: Avulsed teeth should remain splinted for no more than 7 to 10 days. This condition warrants the shortest stabilization period, because of the propensity to develop progressive external root replacement-resorption resulting in ankylosis. Permitting physiologic tooth movement utilizing nonrigid splints seems to deter this process.

Immature teeth with wide open apices have a good potential to revascularize and maintain vitality if replantation is accomplished within 30 minutes. These teeth are carefully observed for radiographic or clinical signs of pulpal degeneration. Radiographs are obtained at 2, 6, and 12 weeks, and semiannually thereafter. Immediate pulp extirpation followed by calcium hydroxide obturation is performed at the first signs of internal or external root resorption or periapical disease.

Mature teeth with closed apices and immature teeth with extended extra-alveolar periods should be pulpectomized 24 to 48 hours after replantation, and left unmedicated. At splint removal 7 to 10 days after injury, calcium hydroxide obturation short of the radiographic apex is performed. Reapplication of calcium hydroxide should be considered at 3 weeks if radiographic evidence of lack of obturation exists, and subsequently at intervals of 2 to 3 months for the first year. Radiographs are made at each obturation visit. Final conventional endodontic obturation can be considered after 1 year if transient external root resorption has resolved.

The anticipated complication of replanted teeth is progressive replacement-resorption and development of ankylosis. In the young growing patient, ankylosis will result in severe infraocclusion of the replanted tooth, and a significant alveolar bone defect if extraction is delayed. Evidence of developing ankylosis should prompt consideration of extraction to prevent prosthetic complications. Because of the nature of avulsion injuries and the multitude of variables that can affect a successful outcome, multiple complications can be anticipated. When the clinician recognizes declining prognostic indicators, such as ankylosis and irreversible root replacement-resorption, definitive action to end the treatment course is taken. Prosthetic rehabilitation is a viable alternative to a long and arduous treatment course when the physiologic response is unfavorable.

F. Alveolar fracture

Alveolar fracture is an extremely common complication of injury to the permanent dentition. By definition, any fracture of the alveolar bone results when a tooth is significantly luxated or avulsed. The diagnosis of alveolar fracture must be considered if concomitant dental luxation or avulsion is present. Treatment is directed at the primary traumatic defect, and in the case of dental avulsion or luxation, the alveolar component is often a secondary diagnosis.

The existence of a comminuted alveolar fracture will have a negative impact on the prognosis of avulsed or luxated teeth. Treatment is directed primarily at the alveolar fracture when segments of alveolar bone and associated teeth are fractured en bloc. If clinical and radiographic examination confirms the integrity of the alveolar socket, treatment should be directed toward bone-to-bone union. This is contrary to treatment objectives in managing dental avulsions and luxations where the primary goal is to encourage healing of the periodontium.

1. **Diagnosis:** Diagnosis of an alveolar fracture has a significant impact on treatment, particularly when there is concomitant dental luxation or avulsion. By definition, an intrusive or lateral dental luxation will result in fracture of the alveolar bone. In intrusive injuries the floor of the alveolar socket is penetrated. Lateral luxation generally results in labial cortical plate fracture, although lingual and interdental alveolar fractures may occur. In the case of dental extrusion or avulsion, the necessary expansion of the alveolar process to permit exarticulation may also result in alveolar fracture. In any case, an empirical diagnosis of alveolar fracture can be made. Radiographic confirmation may not be definitive.

   Occasionally an en bloc segment of alveolus, including multiple teeth, will be fractured. The teeth within the fracture are intact, denoting a segmental dentoalveolar injury. This diagnosis can be made by clinical inspection and manipulation of the injured segment.

2. **Treatment:** When the primary diagnosis is dental

avulsion or luxation, treatment should be directed at this injury. Potential problems arise when the alveolus is significantly fractured or comminuted, making nonrigid stabilization difficult. In such situations, reduction of the injury is the primary focus, perhaps requiring a more rigid or invasive splint for stabilization. In segmental dentoalveolar fractures with no associated tooth mobility a more rigid type of splinting is acceptable. A general guide is to use the least rigid form of splinting necessary for reduction.

3. **Complications:** Alveolar fractures generally have a very good prognosis, since the objective is to obtain bone-to-bone union. This is easily accomplished with 2 to 6 weeks of stabilization, depending on the extent of the injury. Few complications of alveolar bone fractures can be anticipated. Problems may arise if the alveolar fracture is a major component of an avulsion or luxation. In these cases, extended therapy should be directed at management of the dental component of the injury. Treatment modifications may include the need for rigid or more invasive splinting regimens and extended periods of stabilization. It may be necessary therefore to extend the period of stabilization when a significant comminuted alveolar bone fracture exists, although this may have a negative effect on the dental component of the injury.

Evaluation of alveolar fractures and devising pragmatic and effective treatment to deal with these complex situations requires knowledge and thought. Treatment includes splinting to reduce the fracture and an extended period of stabilization. In general, 4 to 6 weeks can be considered the maximum period of time for stabilization of any alveolar fracture. Prolonged stabilization is viewed in light of the potential complications that may result from prolonged splinting.

BIBLIOGRAPHY

Andreasen JO: Luxation injuries, in *Traumatic Injuries of the Teeth*. Philadelphia, WB Saunders, 1981.

Andreasen JO: Treatment of fractured and avulsed teeth. *J Am Dent Assoc* 1971; 97:29–48.

Antrim DD, Bakland LK, Parker MW: Treatment of endodontic urgent care cases. *Dent Clin North Am* 1986; 30:549–572.

Castaldi CR: Sports related oral and facial injuries in the young athlete: A new challenge for the pediatric dentist. *Pediatr Dent* 1986; 8:311–316.

Croll TP, Pascon EA, Langeland K: Traumatically injured primary incisors: A clinical and histiologic study. *J Dent Child* 1987; 54:401–422.

Davis NJ: Management of traumatic dental injuries in children. *NY State Dent J* 1988; 54:22–24.

Dean JA, Avery DR, Swartz ML: Attachment of anterior tooth fragments. *Pediatr Dent* 1986; 8:139–143.

Durr DP, Sveen OB: Pulpal responses after the avulsion and replantation of permanent teeth. *J Pedodont* 1987; 11:301–310.

Fuks AB, Bielak S, Chosak A: Clinical and radiographic assessment of direct pulp capping and pulpotomy. *Pediatr Dent* 1981; 4:240–244.

Garon MW, Merkle A, Wright JT: Mouth protectors and oral trauma: A study of adolescent football players. *J Am Dent Assoc* 1986; 112:662–663.

Garrett GB: Forced eruption in the treatment of transverse root fractures. *J Am Dent Assoc* 1985; 111:270–272.

Gazit E, Sarnat H, Lieberman M: Timing of orthodontic tooth movement in a case with traumatized and avulsed anterior teeth. *J Dent Child* 1988; 55:304–311.

Joho JP, Marechaux SC: Trauma in the primary dentition: A clinical presentation. *J Dent Child* 1980; 47:167–174.

Kehoe JC: Splinting and replantation after traumatic avulsion. *J Am Dent Assoc* 1986; 112:224–230.

Kopel HM, Johnson R: Examination and neurologic assessment of children with facial trauma. *Endodont Dent Traumatol* 1985; 1:155–159.

Kruger GO: *Textbook of Oral Surgery*. St Louis, CV Mosby, 1974.

Levine BC, Sadowsky D: Management of an avulsed central incisor: An unusual approach. *Gen Dent* Jan-Feb 1982; 62–63.

McDonald RE, Avery DR, Lynch TR: *Dentistry for the Child and Adolescent.* St Louis, CV Mosby, 1987, pp 512–572.

Maestrello-deMoya MG, Primosch RE: Orofacial trauma and mouth-protector wear among high school varsity basketball players. *J Dent Child* 1989; 56:36–39.

Meadow D, Lindner G, Needleman H: Oral trauma in children. *Pediatr Dent* 1984; 6:248–251.

Moss SJ, Maccaro H: Examination, evaluation and behavior management following injury to primary incisors. *NY State Dent J* 1985; 51:87–92.

Nazif NM, Ross PJ, Webb MD: Intrabony tooth injuries: Reports of two cases. *J Dent Child* 1989; 56:65–68.

Neaverth EJ, Goerig AC: Technique and rationale for splinting. *J Am Dent Assoc* 1980; 100:56–75.

Saad AY: Calcium hydroxide and apexogenesis. *Oral Surg Oral Med Oral Pathol* 1988; 66:499–501.

Seals RR Jr, Morrow RM, Kuebker WA, et al: An evaluation of mouthguard programs in Texas high school football. *J Am Dent Assoc* 1985; 110:904–909.

Sonis AL: Longitudinal study of discolored primary teeth and effect on succedaneous teeth. *J Pediatr* 1987; 11:247–252.

Spalding PM, Fields HW, Torney D, et al: The changing role of endodontics and orthodontics in the management of traumatically intruded permanent incisors. *Pediatr Dent* 1985; 7:104–110.

Wald CY: Consequences of intrusive injuries to primary teeth. *J Pedodont* 1978; 2:67–77.

Zilberman Y, et al: Effect of trauma to primary incisors on root development of their permanent successors. *Pediatr Dent* 1986; 8:289–293.

Chapter 4 _____

The Medically Compromised Patient

Francis B. Olsen

_____

The objectives of management of the medically compromised patient are to form a treatment plan that takes into consideration the potential complications due to the disease, and to provide a level of care that both enhances the patient's quality of life and does not inadvertently cause any harm.

Many medically compromised patients live with systemic breakdown adequately controlled via the advancements in medical technology and current therapy, which can prolong and maintain an acceptable quality of life.

I. **PATIENT ASSESSMENT AND DATA COLLECTION**
   The major goals of patient assessment and data collection are:
   1. **Identification of systemic disorders** that may affect dental treatment, and vice versa
   2. **Protection of clinician, staff, and other patients** from infectious disease processes that could be acquired or transmitted during dental treatment
   3. **Development of a patient profile** that results in a productive discussion between the dentist and treating physician
   4. **Medicolegal identification** of processes for which dental treatment may have an adverse effect and ultimately place the clinician at risk for legal action

II. **CARDIAC DISEASE**
   A. **Murmur**
      1. **Definition/description:** Murmurs are sounds caused by turbulence in the circulation to the valves and chambers of the heart. Murmurs can be functional or organic. Functional murmurs are sounds caused by turbulence and are not associated with organic heart damage; organic murmurs are sounds caused

by a pathologic abnormality of the heart. Functional murmurs are often present during childhood and disappear at the onset of adolescence. A second form of functional murmur is acquired by women during pregnancy, but disappears after delivery and leaves no residual problem.

2. **Clinical presentation/symptoms:** Patients with mitral valve regurgitation present most commonly with dyspnea. Cardiac output diminishes later in the disease. Patients often become easily fatigued. Mitral valve prolapse is characterized by systolic clicks and a late systolic murmur. The condition may affect as many as 17% of the population.

    Other conditions of significance are mitral stenosis, aortic stenosis, aortic regurgitation, and tricuspid and pulmonic valve disease.

3. **Dental therapy:** The major consideration in patients with murmur is prevention of infectious endocarditis. A history of a possible murmur should be investigated and substantiated by consultation with the patient's physician. Patients with a documented organic murmur require antibiotic prophylaxis as recommended by the American Heart Association (dated 1990) before dental treatment that may induce bleeding. Emergency dental treatment may be rendered by giving the patient the appropriate dose of antibiotics 1–2 hours before the anticipated procedure. Ongoing dental therapy includes maintenance of a healthy oral environment, accomplished by regular dental prophylaxis and encouragement of meticulous oral hygiene at home. Treatment may be enhanced with the addition of an oral antimicrobial rinse such as chlorhexidine (Peridex). The patient should also be advised that in the future all dental treatment must be accompanied by proper antibiotic prophylaxis.

B. **Rheumatic heart disease**

1. **Definition/description:** Rheumatic fever is a severe form of streptococcal infection characterized by fever, rash, joint swelling and pain, chorea, and myocarditis. The cardiac damage that results from

an acute attack of rheumatic fever is called rheumatic heart disease, and involves scarring and calcification of the mitral or aortic valve, which may result in stenosis or regurgitation.

2. **Clinical presentation/symptoms:** The major manifestations of rheumatic fever are arthritis, carditis, chorea, erythema marginatum, and subcutaneous nodules. The arthritis associated with rheumatic fever develops rapidly and lasts for approximately 2 to 3 weeks. Erythema marginatum is a nonpruritic skin rash that occurs in about 5% of patients. Subcutaneous nodules are firm, painless, colorless, subcutaneous swellings, also seen in 5% of patients. Carditis associated with rheumatic fever reveals itself clinically as an abnormal murmur, pericardial rub, cardiac enlargement, congestive heart failure, or a combination of these symptoms. The incidence of significant cardiac damage following the initial attack of rheumatic fever varies from 30% to 80%. The erythrocyte sedimentation rate usually increases, and there is elevation of the antistreptolysin titer.

3. **Dental therapy:** If the patient's medical history suggests the possibility of a childhood febrile infection with joint pain, the possibility of existing rheumatic heart disease must be ruled out. Consultation with the patient's physician is urged. If rheumatic heart disease is present, antibiotic prophylaxis must be used before any dental manipulation.

C. **Congenital heart disease**

1. **Definition/description:** Some form of cardiovascular development or defect occurs in 9 of 1,000 births. Causes of congenital heart disease include rubella syndrome and fetal alcohol syndrome. The major congenital heart disease defects include atrial and ventricular septal defects, patent ductus arteriosus, transposition of the great arteries, persistent truncus arteriosus, tetralogy of Fallot, pulmonary stenosis, and coarctation of the aorta.

2. **Clinical presentation/symptoms:** The clinical consequences of congenital cardiac defects depend on

the type and severity of the defect. Cyanosis, hypoxic episodes, polycythemia, and congestive heart failure are consequences of right-to-left shunts and are usually recognized in childhood. Atrial septal defects may remain asymptomatic until adulthood, when right-to-left shunting, atrial arrhythmia, cardiac failure, or pulmonary hypertension may develop. A universal consequence of congenital heart disease is a predisposition to infectious endocarditis.

3. **Dental therapy:** Treatment considerations for patients with certain congenital heart diseases do not differ from those with other cardiovascular diseases. An ambulatory patient with congenital impairment may display little physical evidence of underlying disease. There is risk of infection that could potentiate infective endocarditis, heart failure, and a variety of congenital arrhythmias. The clinician should maintain careful consultative support from the patient's physician.

D. **Heart valve replacement**
   1. **Definition/description:** The causes of valvular disease have been discussed. Patients with significant disability are surgically treated with prosthetic valve replacement.
   2. **Dental therapy:** The main considerations of dental therapy after medical management of valvular disease are (1) prevention of infectious endocarditis and (2) special care for the patient receiving anticoagulant therapy, who is at great risk for bleeding after surgical procedures. Consultation with the patient's physician will establish the proper antibiotic protocol and aid in the management of the anticoagulant therapy. The level of anticoagulation is monitored using the prothrombin time (PT). Since sodium warfarin (Coumadin) is a vitamin K antagonist and interferes with the synthesis of coagulation factors II, VII, IX, and X by the liver, its effects may be reversed by the administration of vitamin K. Verification of the patient's coagulation potential can be done by establishing that PT is within one

and one-half times the normal limit. The potential for bleeding should be evaluated by the nature of the procedure. Adjustment of warfarin dosage should be done in consultation with the patient's physician. Recent literature suggests that a higher PT (up to two times control) may be acceptable in minor surgical procedures.

One goal of dental therapy for the patient being prepared for valve replacement is to identify and eliminate actual and potential sources of orofacial infection that could infect prosthetic material implanted into the heart or great vessels. The patient is questioned regarding swellings, foul taste, drainage, gingival bleeding, or pressure or temperature sensitivity localized to the oral cavity. Periodontal examination will reveal any areas of fluctuance or drainage, carious lesions, tender or mobile teeth, and mucosal lesions or irritation. A radiographic survey is performed to rule out bone and periapical disease and the level of periodontal support. Other goals of dental therapy are to establish an optimal level of oral hygiene, restore teeth that are repairable, and remove periodontally or periapically involved teeth. Teeth with a questionable prognosis should be removed before cardiac surgery. The patient is prepared in consultation with the physician and the use of appropriate antibiotic prophylaxis. An oral antimicrobial rinse such as chlorhexidine (Peridex) can be used before surgery. After treatment has been rendered and the patient is deemed free of orofacial sources of infection, an oral antimicrobial rinse can be used indefinitely. The patient is instructed to maintain meticulous oral hygiene and to be aware of the risk factors of orofacial infection and the potential for injury to cardiac valves. The patient is dentally evaluated regularly and given the appropriate support to maintain a healthy environment.

E. Angina pectoris

    1. Definition/description: Angina pectoris is a form of symptomatic ischemic heart disease produced when myocardial demands exceed the ability of the coronary arteries to deliver oxygen. A prime cause of angina is atherosclerotic heart disease with obstruction of one or more of the three major coronary arteries. It can also be produced from excess oxygen demand, limited oxygen carrying capacity of the blood due to anemia, or inadequate perfusion by the coronary arteries during a hypotensive episode.

2. **Clinical presentation/symptoms:** Angina is often precipitated by emotional stress or physical exertion and is relieved by rest. The patient typically shows signs of anxiety during an attack and is unable to localize the source of the discomfort. The pain is described as a heavy sensation and can radiate to the shoulders, arms, or mandible. It is usually brief.

3. **Dental therapy:** Patients with stable angina and who have not experienced myocardial infarction are at much lower risk for dental complications during therapy than patients with unstable angina. Good rapport with the patient can reduce levels of anxiety. Dental appointments should be short, and nitroglycerine should be available. When appropriate sedative techniques are to be used and if the patient is significantly compromised, hospitalization for dental treatment should be considered.

F. **Myocardial infarction**

1. **Definition/description:** Myocardial infarction is the result of prolonged ischemic injury to the heart, particularly subsequent to progressive coronary artery disease. Other causes of myocardial ischemia include spasms of the coronary arteries and vasculitic involvement of the coronary arteries.

2. **Clinical presentation/symptoms:** The patient usually has severe chest pain, which may radiate to the left arm or jaw and is associated with shortness of breath, palpitations, nausea, and vomiting. Although described as similar to that of angina, the pain is more severe and protracted. The patient appears diaphoretic and in acute distress, often with

what has been described as a fearful look. Diagnosis is confirmed with electrocardiographic and enzyme studies. Complications may include arrhythmias and congestive heart failure.

3. **Dental therapy:** Vital signs are taken and documented at each dental visit. The clinician must categorize postmyocardial patients into three groups: (1) those with a recent infarct, that is, within 6 months, for which the physician is continuing stablization of postinfarct complications and symptoms; (2) patients with infarct more than 6 months previously but who continue to have symptoms, such as angina, arrhythmias, or congestive failure; and (3) patients with an old infarct without symptoms. Patients in group 1 have the highest risk for subsequent infarction. Consultation with the patient's physician is essential. All elective dental procedures are deferred until cardiovascular complications are stabilized. Group 2 patients are at reduced risk, yet significant precautions must be taken. Routine dental procedures may be performed. Group 3 patients are at the same risk as other patients with ischemic heart disease. These patients should be given short appointments, in an environment developed to minimize stress. Pain control is important, and the use of a local anesthetic including the judicious use of epinephrine 1:100,000 may be indicated. Decision to premedicate with nitroglycerin is made in conjunction with the patient's physician. Adjunct therapy such as inhalation analgesia can be used after consultation.

III. ARRHYTHMIA

1. **Definition/description:** Arrhythmia is disturbance of the normal rhythm of the heart. It may be a manifestation of underlying atherosclerotic heart disease, and may be exacerbated during stress and anxiety. Arrhythmia of significant magnitude may increase the risk for angina, myocardial infarction, congestive heart failure, transient ischemic attacks, and cerebral vascular accident.

2. **Clinical presentation/symptoms:** Cardiac arrhyth-

mia may be asymptomatic and detected because of a change in the rate or rhythm of the pulse, for example, slow pulse (bradycardia) or fast pulse (tachycardia). Symptoms that suggest the presence of arrhythmia include dizziness, fatigue, congestive heart failure, angina, and most serious, cardiac arrest. Electrocardiograms and cardiac catheterization are useful in detecting and identifying arrhythmia.

3. **Dental therapy:** Stress avoidance is crucial in the treatment of these patients. Patients with arrhythmia are at risk for serious complications including cardiac arrest. Consultation with the patient's physician is required to establish the nature of the arrhythmia and its stability. Patients receive short morning appointments and may be given nitrous oxide–oxygen inhalation analgesia. Avoid using epinephrine, because it can precipitate a life-threatening arrhythmia in a susceptible patient. Epinephrine is not used in gingival retraction or directly to control bleeding. With these precautions, patients with arrhythmia can receive comprehensive dental treatment.

IV. CONGESTIVE HEART FAILURE

1. **Definition/description:** Congestive heart failure is defined as the inability of the heart to deliver an adequate supply of blood to meet metabolic demands. It may involve failure of the right or left ventricle or both. Etiologic factors include essential hypertension, cardiac valvular disease, and chronic atherosclerotic heart disease. Congestive heart failure is associated with a mortality rate of approximately 50% within 5 years, and patients have increased morbidity and mortality with stress.

2. **Clinical presentation/symptoms:** Patients with congestive heart failure have shortness of breath and dyspnea, particularly on exertion. These symptoms may be exacerbated when the patient is lying flat (orthopnea), and patients report sleeping with several pillows. Shortness of breath can cause the patient to wake at night with paroxysmal nocturnal dyspnea. These symptoms are pathognomonic of

left-sided heart failure. Failure of the right side of
the heart includes right upper abdominal discomfort
due to hepatic congestion and peripheral edema.
3. **Dental therapy:** The most important consideration
in dental management in patients with congestive
heart failure is to minimize stress. Limit treatment
to short morning appointments, and consider the
use of adjunct sedation. Patients may not be comfortable in the supine position during treatment. The
patient should be monitored verbally during treatment. If the patient becomes fatigued the appointment should be terminated and rescheduled. Patients taking digoxin are susceptible to arrythmia,
and all precautions should be enforced. Patients
taking digoxin also are susceptible to nausea and
vomiting.

V. HYPERTENSION

1. **Definition/description:** Hypertension has been defined as a condition wherein a supine adult has a
resting arterial pressure of 160 mm Hg systolic and
95 mm Hg diastolic, or higher. In the United States
approximately 60 million persons have hypertension: 35 million with definite hypertension and 25
million with borderline hypertension. The disorder
can be divided into two major categories: essential
or idiopathic hypertension, found in 90% of the
cases, and secondary hypertension, caused by renal
and adrenal disease.
2. **Clinical presentation/symptoms:** Most patients
with hypertension are asymptomatic, and discovery
is made on routine examination or screening. When
symptoms are present the most common is headache, manifest on awakening in the morning and
disappearing during the day. Patients experience
dizziness, fatigue, and palpitations, and in severe
cases weakness, blurred vision, and epistaxis. If left
untreated, hypertension can lead to cerebral vascular accident, renal disease, and coronary artery disease.
3. **Dental therapy:** A blood pressure level is recorded
at the first visit, and if evidence of hypertension is

seen the patient is referred for assessment and management before dental therapy. The patient with a dental emergency is offered palliative therapy to relieve pain or to control bleeding or infection, after telephone consultation with the patient's physician. If the patient's physician is not available, prudent judgment must be made to provide short-term relief of the dental problem. Adequate time invested at the consultation to establish good rapport with the patient is the first step in alleviating patient stress, thus helping to avoid rapid rise in blood pressure and a serious physiologic problem. Short appointments, sedative therapy if needed, and good pain control are necessary to keep anxiety levels down. Judicious use of local anesthetic with epinephrine is recommended to maintain adequate pain control. Familiarity with the hypertension medication prescribed permits the clinician to be knowledgeable of potential side effects. Patients who experience xerostomia should receive aggressive care, including counselling regarding diet, oral hygiene, home care, and in severe cases adjunctive topical fluoride therapy. At the end of each appointment restore the dental chair to the upright position slowly to prevent dizziness associated with orthostatic hypotension, and have the patient sit quietly for 2 or 3 minutes before arising to leave the operatory.

VI. PULMONARY DISEASE/CHRONIC OBSTRUCTIVE PULMONARY DISEASE

1. **Definition/description:** The two most common forms of chronic obstructive pulmonary disease (COPD) are emphysema and chronic bronchitis. These are characterized by obstruction of air flow during respiratory efforts. Emphysema is defined as distention of the air spaces distal to the terminal bronchiole, with destruction of the alveolar septum. Chronic bronchitis is defined as a condition associated with excessive tracheal bronchial mucus production sufficient to cause cough, and expectoration for 3 months of the year for more than 2 consecutive years. The two forms often coexist. The most

important etiologic factors in COPD are cigarette smoking and chronic exposure to occupational environmental pollutants.

2. **Clinical presentation/symptoms:** The clinical signs and symptoms of chronic bronchitis and emphysema are frequently indistinct. Patients with chronic bronchitis have chronic cough with copious sputum production, and are overweight and cyanotic; patients with emphysema have a minimal, nonproductive cough. Patients with bronchitis have elevated PCO_2 and decreased PO_2, leading to erythrocytosis and elevated hematocrit; those with emphysema have relatively normal PCO_2 and decreased PO_2 and maintain normal hemoglobin saturation. Patients with COPD become dyspneic to the point of debilitation, and are susceptible to recurrent pulmonary infections. Pulmonary hypertension can lead to cor pulmonale, right-sided heart failure, and ultimately emphysema that is irreversible and incurable.

3. **Dental therapy:** Patients with COPD have compromised respiratory function; therefore any depression of respiration should be avoided. Patients should be placed in upright chair position for treatment. Local anesthetic may be used judiciously; however, bilateral block is contraindicated because of the potential of inducing a choking sensation. Rubber dam is to be avoided because patients with COPD may feel their air supply is compromised. Both narcotics and barbiturates cause respiratory depression and should be avoided. Patients taking corticosteroids may require supplementation if they are to be placed under any physiologic stress. All drug therapy should be coordinated via consultation with the patient's physician.

A. **Asthma**

1. **Definition/description:** Asthma is a syndromic disease consisting of dyspnea, cough, and wheezing. During an asthma attack the bronchi and bronchioles are occluded by thick mucous plugs, leading to decreased diameter of the airway.

   A variety of disorders can result from asthma,

including immunologic abnormalities that cause inhaled antigens to trigger a hypersensitivity response. Asthma may be induced by aspirin ingestion. Allergic asthma is called extrinsic asthma; idiosyncratic asthma is referred to as intrinsic asthma. Emotional stress is implicated in some patients with asthma. A small percentage of patients develop status asthmaticus, which is a severe, prolonged asthmatic attack refractory to usual therapy.

2. **Clinical presentation/symptoms:** Asthma is characterized by sudden onset of tightness in the chest and cough. Respirations are difficult, and there is expiratory wheeze. The episodes are usually self-limiting and end with a productive cough.

3. **Dental therapy:** A careful history will identify whether the asthma is allergic or nonallergic, and the precipitating factors, frequency and severity of attacks, and how they are managed. The patient should be questioned regarding the number of times emergency room care was needed. A list of all medications the patient is taking is compiled. Consultation with the patient's physician is necessary in the case of patients who have severe asthma. Advise the patient to bring the medication to each appointment, particularly any type of inhalant medication. Avoid giving aspirin or aspirin-containing products, nonsteroidal anti-inflammatory drugs, barbiturates, and narcotics. The patient taking a corticosteroid may require supplemental dosage when subjected to physiologic stress. Efforts should be made to reduce the patient's level of anxiety, for example, with judicious use of nitrous oxide–oxygen inhalation or small doses of diazepam.

B. **Tuberculosis**

1. **Definition/description:** The causative agent in tuberculosis is *Mycobacterium tuberculosis,* an obligate aerobe that requires an atmosphere of high oxygen tension. Typical mode of transmission is by way of infected airborne droplets of mucus or saliva that have been expelled from the lungs during coughing.

2. **Clinical presentation/symptoms:** Patients are normally examined because of a history of exposure to tuberculosis, a positive skin test for tuberculosis, or radiographic findings. Patients may have fever, chills, night sweats, productive cough, and weight loss. It is most common for a patient to present with a positive tuberculin skin test but not active infection. The presence of active pulmonary disease is usually confirmed by examination of the sputum.

3. **Dental therapy:** For all patients with a history of tuberculosis, consultation with the patient's physician is required to establish the presence of active infection. Patients with a positive sputum culture should not be treated in the outpatient environment. Some patients may present with an oral manifestation of the disease, commonly an ulcer on the dorsum of the tongue. Cervical and submandibular lymph nodes can be infected, and are usually enlarged and painful and may form draining abscesses.

VII. **END-STAGE RENAL DISEASE**

1. **Definition/description:** End-stage renal disease is defined as bilateral progressive and chronic deterioration of nephrons, resulting in uremia and finally in death. Causative factors include nephrosclerosis secondary to hypertension, diabetic neuropathy, hyaline nephritis, and drug-induced nephrotoxicity. Function is maintained until approximately 50% of the nephrons are destroyed. As the disease progresses, patients manifest azotemia, anemia, changes in white blood cells that lead to alteration of immune inflammatory responses and ultimately greater susceptibility to infection, and tendencies toward hemorrhage related to abnormal platelet aggregation and decreased platelet factor III. There are also changes in bone metabolism, leading to osteomalacia, osteitis fibrosa, and osteosclerosis.

2. **Clinical presentation/symptoms:** Patients with renal failure are easily fatigued, appear weak, and often have anorexia, nausea, vomiting, and a pruritis that may be associated with brownish yellow

spots caused by retention of carotene-like pigments normally excreted by the kidney. Cardiovascular involvement includes hypertension and congestive heart failure. It is not uncommon for patients to have bleeding disorders, seen as petechiae or ecchymoses on the skin or mucous membranes.

3. **Dental therapy:** The goal of dental therapy is to provide and maintain a healthy oral environment. Consultation with a physician will provide information regarding the status of renal function. When treating patients undergoing renal dialysis, rigorous infection control procedures must be observed. Patients should be appointed for treatment on days when they are not receiving dialysis, because of the use of heparin as an anticoagulant. Patients with shunts should receive appropriate antibiotic prophylaxis to prevent end arteritis. If any oral or periodontal surgery is contemplated, a coagulation and bleeding profile should be obtained. Tetracyclines are contraindicated for antibiotic therapy, as are aspirin or nonsteroidal anti-inflammatory drugs for pain control.

VIII. **LIVER DISEASE**
   A. **Hepatitis**
      1. **Definition/description:** Hepatitis, an inflammatory disease of the liver, may be caused by numerous factors. The major concern for dentists is related to viral hepatitis, including hepatitis A, hepatitis B, non-A non-B hepatitis (type C), and delta hepatitis (type D). During the acute infection there is necrosis of liver cells and generalized inflammatory response throughout the entire hepatic lobule. Hepatitis A, which was traditionally referred to as infectious hepatitis, is transmitted primarily by the fecal-oral route. Most patients recover without residual problems and are not carriers. Hepatitis B is transmitted by parenteral, venereal, and vertical or mother-to-child modes. The hepatitis B patient carries a 10% risk of remaining a carrier. In these patients there is surface antigenemia and the disease remains infectious. Non-A non-B hepatitis is a di-

agnosis primarily of exclusion. Patients show no antigenic markers, with elevated liver enzyme test results. In many of these patients the disorder progresses to chronic active hepatitis. Delta hepatitis is a severe form of hepatitis requiring hepatitis B carrier status as a cofactor for infection. This severe fulminating form of hepatitis is associated with high morbidity and mortality.

2. **Clinical presentation/symptoms:** Many patients are unaware that they have hepatitis B at the time of infection. Symptoms have been described as flu-like with concomitant nausea and vomiting, low-grade fever, and loss of appetite. Jaundice is evident when serum bilirubin level reaches 3 mg/dL plasma. Laboratory testing will show increased levels of hepatic alanine aminotransferase (ALT; previously SGPT), aspartate aminotransferase (AST; SGOT), and LDH enzymes. The presence of a surface antigenemia is appreciated most commonly in type B hepatitis and in delta hepatitis.

    Medical management of hepatitis is primarily supportive. Its goal is to allow the patient to recover by minimizing liver function. Other measures are preventive and relate to controlling transmission of the disease to family members and others in close contact with the patient. Hyperimmune globulin or vaccination are usually used as prophylaxis.

3. **Dental therapy:** It is important to establish which form of hepatitis the patient had and whether there is residual disease. This information can be obtained by consultation with the patient's physician and a hepatitis laboratory screen including liver function tests (ALT, AST, lactic dehydrogenase [LDH]), presence of hepatitis-related antigens, or hepatitis antibody titer (Table 4–1). If there is no evidence of hepatitis infection in either an active or carrier state and no liver dysfunction, normal dental treatment can be performed without further consideration. In the patient with active liver disease or residual liver defect three considerations must be dealt with. If surgical procedures are being planned,

TABLE 4–1.

Hepatitis B Serologic Panel

HBsAs	Surface antigen
HBsAb	Surface antibody
HBcAb	Core antibody
HBeAg	e antigen
HBeAb	e antibody

the clinician must be aware of the patient's coagulation profile; this can be done by testing prothrombin time. Second, depending on the severity of dysfunction, the clinician must be aware of all pharmacologic agents that are metabolized by the liver that may be required by the patient. If necessary, dosage accommodations or changes in medication should be made. The third consideration is infection control. Since it has become clear that all patients who present risk of disease transmission cannot be routinely identified, rigorous adherence to Centers for Disease Control (CDC) barrier standards and American Dental Association (ADA) guidelines for sterilization must be maintained. In addition, all clinical staff with patient contact or involved in instrumentation should receive hepatitis B vaccine.

B. Cirrhosis

1. **Definition/description:** Cirrhosis relates to chronic destruction of liver cells and concomitant and progressive scarring as a result of protracted insult to the liver. A leading cause of cirrhosis is chronic alcohol abuse. There is progressing diminution of metabolic and excretory functions, leading to total hepatic failure. This degeneration ultimately affects the liver's ability to synthesize protein, albumin, lipoproteins, and of importance, clotting factors. In addition there is impaired ability to detoxify drugs and other substances.

2. **Clinical presentation/symptoms:** Often cirrhosis is not clinically detectable but is found at autopsy. There is no clear-cut definition as to the amount of alcoholic intake that will produce cirrhosis, but data

suggest that the person who consumes one pint of whiskey per day or its equivalent for 10 years will have cirrhotic signs and symptoms. Often the clinician is alerted to an alcohol problem by patient history or by a family member. Repeated detection of alcohol on breath suggests alcoholism. Clinically, alcohol abuse produces physical signs such as spider angiomas, palmar erythema, and peripheral edema. As liver damage progresses ascites and portal hypertension develop. Portal hypertension ultimately may produce esophageal varices and place the patient at risk for a serious hemorrhagic event. Laboratory testing of liver enzymes will show large increases in ALT, AST, and alkaline phosphatase levels. Microcytic anemia may be found secondary to vitamin B_{12} and folate deficiency. A coagulation profile study will reveal increased PT, decreased platelet count, and increased bleeding time. Because of the associated metabolic alterations serum albumin concentration is elevated.

3. **Dental therapy:** The role of dental therapy in the care of the patient with alcoholism or resultant alcoholic cirrhosis is multiple. Many of these patients suffer chronic oral neglect, and as a result may seek care during a period of acute pain or infection. Until the patient is medically stable, palliative care is provided to relieve pain and to control infection or bleeding. Because of the debilitated state of the liver, the clinician must have an awareness of drugs metabolized by the liver or that may exacerbate existing bleeding problems. Aspirin-containing drugs and nonsteroidal anti-inflammatory drugs are contraindicated. Once the alcholic patient makes a commitment to optimal oral health, the dentist and the care delivered will provide a significant contribution in restoring the patient's self-image. Dental care must also include monitoring the patient for any of the known head and neck malignancies associated with alcohol abuse, especially in conjunction with tobacco use. The clinician can counsel the patient about the potential for these diseases and en-

hance the patient's motivation to continue to abstain from using alcohol and tobacco. If the patient's care includes extensive surgical procedures, a decision must be made in conjunction with the patient's physician as to whether a hospital is the appropriate environment for care, especially if there is need for transfusion of platelets or fresh frozen plasma. During therapy these patients require strong emotional support and good pain control. These patients may metabolize local anesthestics at a significantly higher rate than normal. Sedatives and tranquilizers should be used only after consultation with the patient's physician.

IX. PREGNANCY AND LACTATION

1. **Definition/description:** Although pregnancy is not a compromised medical state, it presents some problems to the clinician. The pregnant woman manifests many physiologic changes. Hormone production changes in order to preserve viability of the fetus and prepare the breast for lactation. Flow murmur, which is a functional murmur, can be detected in many pregnant women. Hemodynamic changes include increased maternal blood volume to compensate for the needs of the developing fetus. Respiratory rate also increases.

2. **Clinical presentation/symptoms:** Most women may suspect that they are pregnant after they have missed a menstrual cycle. There may be nausea and breast tenderness. Physicians usually test urine for the presence of human chorionic gonadotropin (hCG), which in conjunction with other clinical findings may suggest pregnancy. Further serum testing of hCG is necessary for confirmation.

3. **Dental therapy:** Dental care for the pregnant woman is primarily preventive. Patients should be advised of the need for meticulous home care. Oral prophylaxis may be performed at the end of the first trimester and again at the start of the third trimester. Because of hormonal effects on vasculature some patients appear to be at risk for "pregnancy gingivitis," which may manifest as an exuberant

form of gingival inflammation. Effects of this condition can be minimized with appropriate home care. All elective dental treatment should be deferred until after delivery of the child. Emergent care can be delivered during the second trimester; before this, palliative treatment should be attempted. Most drugs used in oral health care delivery, including lidocaine, penicillin, and erythromycin, have shown no harm to the developing fetus and can be used judiciously. Drugs that are absolutely contraindicated include tetracycline, diazepam, and nitrous oxide. Treatment in the pregnant woman requires an understanding of the balance between the need for dental treatment and the risk to the fetus. These are suggested guidelines, but clearly all treatment should be rendered in consultation with the patient's obstetrician.

X. SEIZURE DISORDERS

1. **Definition/description:** Three major seizure disorders are of concern to the clinician. The most common is grand mal seizure, characterized by abrupt loss of consciousness and clonic contractions of the muscles of the extremities that may last as long as 5 minutes. Patients are usually disoriented and confused for a time after the seizure (postictal phase). Petit mal seizures are characterized by loss of consciousness for a very short time (no more than 30 seconds), without any motor dysfunction. Patients may suddenly lose contact and stare aimlessly, but may resume normal activity without being aware that a seizure has taken place. Psychomotor seizures involve no loss of consciousness but are characterized by bizarre behavior.

2. **Clinical presentation/symptoms:** The signs and symptoms of seizure disorder are described above. Patients are initially examined to determine the underlying cause of the seizure. Causes may include infection, tumor or abscess, or metabolic imbalance. Some seizure disorders may be corrected by proper medical or surgical intervention. After diagnosis, drug therapy is often initiated to control and

limit seizure activity. The most commonly used drugs are phenytoin (Dilantin), primidone (Mysolene), ethosuximide (Zarontin), carbamazepine (Tegretol), and diazepam (Valium). Phenytoin is no longer considered the drug of choice, because of multiple side effects. In some intractable cases a neurosurgical procedure can be performed on the temporal lobe and has a relatively high success rate in eliminating seizure activity.

3. **Dental therapy:** The patient with a history of seizure disorder should be questioned as to the type of seizure, age at onset, number of seizures per month, time of the most recent seizure, and duration of seizure activity, and current medical regimen used to control seizures. No treatment should be rendered if seizure activity is not under control.

   For those patients who are taking phenytoin, control and management of associated gingival hyperplasia is of major concern. In severe cases, periodontal surgical treatment of hyperplastic tissue is indicated. Aggressive home care and a regular therapeutic and maintenance program is indicated. Consultation with a neurologist to discuss the possibility of replacing phenytoin with a drug that is equally effective in controlling seizures but with minimal gingival side effects may be desirable. A second consideration is prosthetic restoration. Prosthetic care should minimize the use of removable prostheses and porcelain whenever possible.

XI. **CEREBROVASCULAR DISEASE**

1. **Definition/description:** Two critical forms of cerebrovascular disease are of concern. The first is transient ischemic attack (TIA), a short-term reversible neurologic event that may last from 1 minute to 24 hours. If occlusion lasts beyond 24 hours the risk for cerebrovascular accident (CVA) increases. The most significant etiologic factor in cerebrovascular disease is untreated hypertension; however, atherosclerosis and its risk factors, including diabetes mellitus, smoking, and hypercholesterolemia, are

also significant. Oral contraceptive use in women who smoke has been implicated.

2. **Clinical presentation/symptoms:** Most CVAs are preceded by premonitory signs, which may include dizziness, diplopia, motor dysfunction, and changes in speech pattern. Patients may experience sudden unilateral weakness or numbness of the extremities, unilateral visual change, or dizziness, and perhaps may fall. Laboratory tests should include urinalysis, complete blood cell count, erythrocyte sedimentation rate, blood cholesterol levels, and lipid levels. Neuroradiologic procedures, including arteriography, computed tomography, and magnetic resonance imaging, provide data to confirm the diagnosis.

3. **Dental therapy:** When a history of TIA or CVA is noted it is important to ascertain the underlying causes. Consultation with the patient's physician should establish the level of control achieved with prescribed drugs, plus the coagulation profile and any evident concomitant disease, particularly cardiac disorders. Patients should be given short morning appointments; blood pressure should be monitored during the procedure; and use of vasoconstrictor and local anesthetics should be minimal. Agents that do not induce hypotension, such as nitrous oxide–oxygen or small doses of diazepam, may be used to reduce patient stress. Comprehensive dental care can be provided with modification depending on physical disability. If surgical procedures are contemplated, documentation of the coagulation profile with appropriate adjustments made in consultation with the patient's physician should be considered. The patient who has experienced TIA or CVA within 6 months is at high risk for exacerbation, and only palliative treatment should be given until the patient's condition is stable.

XII. **JOINT DISEASE/JOINT REPLACEMENT**

1. **Definition/description:** The three major joint diseases considered are rheumatoid arthritis, osteoarthritis, and gout. Rheumatoid arthritis is a disease

of unknown cause that involves joints symmetrically, particularly the hands and the wrists. Often there are subcutaneous nodules. Onset is in the third or fourth decade of life, and the disease is progressively disabling. Osteoarthritis is the result of breakdown of joint cartilage, often from trauma but usually from aging. Gout is an acute inflammatory arthritis arising from uric acid deposition in the joint space.

2. **Clinical presentation/symptoms:** Rheumatoid arthritis produces pain, swelling, and limitation of joint motion. In long-standing cases joint deformity is observed. Laboratory tests usually show positive rheumatoid factor and elevation of the erythyrocyte sedimentation rate. Positive radiographic findings support the diagnosis. Osteoarthritis may cause enlargement of terminal interphalangeal joints, generalized stiffness, pain, and limitation of range of motion. Laboratory test results are negative for rheumatoid factor, and the erythyrocyte sedimentation rate is normal. Gout produces warm tender joints with severe limitation and range of motion.

3. **Dental therapy:** There are three major areas of concern for the dentist treating a patient with joint disease. A percentage of patients may have disease of the temporomandibular joints, which may affect dental treatment. Second, the medical history should elicit prescribed and nonprescribed medications taken. Patients taking high doses of aspirin are at risk for bleeding due to interference with platelet aggregation. The bleeding abnormalities may last 7 to 10 days after the discontinuation of aspirin therapy. Response to anti-inflammatory drugs may have a similar effect on bleeding profile but with a shorter period of recovery after drug withdrawal. Finally, the patient with a skeletal joint prosthesis may be at risk for late joint infection. This is a controversial area, with little evidence that dental procedures may be responsible for joint infection. Consultation with the orthopedist to determine the most appropriate course of action is warranted. The stan-

dard prophylaxis used to prevent endocarditis is generally appropriate, however. The orthopedist, recognizing the level of risk, may suggest an alternative antibiotic for use in conjunction with the procedure.

XIII. ADRENAL DISEASE

1. **Definition/description:** Hyperfunction of the adrenal medulla can be caused by a tumor called pheochromocytoma. This leads to excessive secretion of epinephrine and norepinephrine. Cushing's syndrome is hyperfunction of the adrenal cortex characterized by the hypersecretion of glucocorticoid hormone. This overactivity can be mediated by diseases that affect the hypothalmus, the anterior pituitary gland, or the adrenal gland itself. Addison's disease represents adrenal gland hypofunction, primarily caused by the destruction of the gland.

2. **Clinical presentation/symptoms:** Patients with pheochromocytoma have headache, palpitations, profuse sweating, and episodic hypertension. Serum concentrations of epinephrine and norepinephrine are elevated. The patient with Cushing's syndrome has characteristic moon facies, obesity, and hirsutism. Hypertension is often present due to fluid retention. Urinary catecholamines, metanephrines, and vanilylmandelic acid levels are elevated. The patient with Addison's disease may experience weakness, weight loss, nausea and vomiting, and orthostatic hypertension. Hyperpigmentation of the buccal and labial mucosa may be noted secondary to increased secretion of adrenocorticotropic hormone (ACTH).

3. **Dental therapy:** Consultation with the patient's physician will establish the level of adrenal suppression and replacement. Major concerns are the patient's reduced capability to deal with stress, and susceptibility to infection and delayed wound healing. If surgical procedures are considered it may be necessary to supplement the patient's steroid dosage. This can be calculated to a level necessary to deal with the anticipated stress. The supplemental

dosage can be reduced to normal over 2 to 3 days. A 7-day course of antibiotic therapy, with either penicillin or erythromycin, can be used to minimize risk for infection. Adjunctive sedation techniques may be used during the procedure to minimize stress. For routine operative or periodontal care major adjustment of the treatment plan may not be necessary.

XIV. DIABETES MELLITUS

1. **Definition/description:** Diabetes mellitus results from an absolute or relative insulin deficiency caused either by low output from the pancreas or by unresponsiveness of peripheral tissues. Although obesity and old age are common risk factors, the most important is heredity. Patients with diabetes are at great risk for vascular, neurologic, and infectious complications, primarily as a result of microcirculatory changes induced by the disease.

   The disease occurs in two forms: insulin-dependent diabetes mellitus (type I) and non-insulin-dependent diabetes mellitus (type II). It should be noted that in some patients type II disease may evolve into type I. It is postulated that autoimmune beta cell destruction occurs slowly in these patients.

2. **Clinical presentation/symptoms:** Symptoms including weight loss, polydypsia, polyuria, and polyphagia should raise the suspicion of diabetes mellitus. Secondary to changes in glucose metabolism are changes in lipid metabolism, leading to increased accumulation of ketones, which may ultimately result in ketoacidosis. This is indicated by polydypsia and polyuria, with nausea and vomiting. In severe cases there may be coma, and ultimately death.

3. **Dental therapy:** Prior to dental treatment in a diabetic patient the level of control must be established. The diabetic patient may have symptoms of other systemic breakdown, including cardiovascular, renal, and peripheral neuropathic changes. Oral complications include generalized rapidly advancing

periodontal disease, candidal infection, and oral mucosal lesions. Routine dental care should be given in the early morning. Patients should be instructed to take the normal dose of insulin and consume a normal meal. They should be monitored during treatment for any signs of hypoglycemia. Sugar should be available in the form of fruit juice or any other easily consumed, rapidly absorbed food. If surgical procedures are contemplated it may be advisable to augment insulin dosage in consultation with the patient's physician and provide prophylactic antibiotic therapy. In patients with an acute infection, consultation with the physician is in order to determine whether an increased dose of insulin is necessary. Penicillin is the drug of choice, and culture and sensitivity testing should be undertaken to establish the presence of other organisms. The report may recommend a change in antibiotic. Patients should be observed daily during treatment of infection until resolution, at which point a physician should examine the patient and establish appropriate insulin dosage. Patients with well-controlled diabetes can receive normal comprehensive dental care.

XV. THYROID DISEASE

1. **Definition/description:** The two major dysfunctions of the thyroid gland are hyperthyroidism and hypothyroidism. The thyroid gland is responsible for the production of thyroxine (T_4), the major regulator of metabolism. Thyroxine also potentiates action of other hormones, including catecholamine and growth hormones. Hyperthyroidism is characterized by increased T_4 production. The converse, insufficient production of thyroid hormone, results in hypothyroidism.

2. **Clinical presentation/symptoms:** Many symptoms of hyperthyroidism reflect metabolic maladjustment. Patients complain of excessive heat and are often nervous, with noticeable tremor, muscle weakness, and diaphoresis. Gastrointestinal symptoms include

increased appetite, diarrhea, and weight loss. Head and neck examination will reveal an enlarged thyroid gland, with the overlying skin very thin and soft. A leading cause of hyperthyroidism is Graves' disease, a putative autoimmune disorder. Older patients may demonstrate hyperthyroidism as a result of multinodular goiter. Diagnosis can be established by documenting the level of T_4 or of triiodothyronine (T_3). Conversely, patients with hypothyroidism complain of weight gain, inability to tolerate cold, and fatigue. Regional examination reveals enlargement of the tongue, puffiness of the face, and dry skin. The diagnosis may be confirmed by evaluating the level of free T_4 and thyroid-stimulating hormone. Primary causes of hypothyroidism include thyroidectomy, Hashimoto's thyroiditis, and previous radioactive iodine therapy.

3. **Dental therapy:** The major concern of therapy is the increased sensitivity to the actions of catecholamines on inadequately treated or untreated hyperthyroidism. Epinephrine as contained in local anesthetic or on gingival retraction cord can precipitate a thyroid storm. This phenomenon is manifested by fever, agitation, and psychotic behavior, and may evolve into life-threatening arrhythmia. The patient with mild hyperthyroidism may experience tachycardia and tremor. Although it is unlikely that a thyrotoxic patient is seen, judicious use of epinephrine may be permitted in the patient with well-controlled hyperthyroidism. (Epinephrine-impregnated cords are not recommended at any time in any patient.) Infections of the orofacial region should be treated aggressively with antibiotic therapy and incision and drainage in conjunction with consultation with the patient's physician. The patient with well-controlled hyperthyroidism can receive comprehensive dental treatment.

Patients with hypothyroidism may have preexisting CNS depression, which can be exacerbated by narcotic analgesics, barbiturates, and tranquilizers. In the patient with well-managed hypothyroidism there are no contraindications to comprehensive general dental care.

XVI. HUMAN IMMUNE DEFICIENCY VIRUS INFECTION

1. **Definition/description:** Human immune deficiency virus (HIV) infection is caused by an RNA retrovirus that attacks primarily the T4 helper lymphocyte and the macrophage. This infection reduces the number of T cells and their immunologic function, making the patient more susceptible to opportunistic infections and certain neoplasms, such as Kaposi's sarcoma and non-Hodgkin's lymphoma.

   HIV-related disease can be divided into four phases. In phase 1 the patient is asymptomatic but tests positive for HIV. Phase 2 is characterized by persistent generalized lymphadenopathy; the patient begins to demonstrate weight loss, night sweats, and diarrhea. In phase 3, or acquired immunodeficiency syndrome (AIDS)–related complex (ARC), the patient may have bouts of minor opportune infections, such as oral candidiasis or the first signs of a malignancy such as Kaposi's sarcoma. Phase 4 is full-blown AIDS; the patient has major opportunistic infection, such as *Pneumocystis carinii* pneumonia.

2. **Clinical presentation/symptoms:** As described, the symptoms of HIV infection are various and progressive. At first patients are asymptomatic but carrying the virus. Subsequently generalized lymphadenopathy develops, with weight loss, night sweats, and diarrhea, followed by minor opportunistic infections and early manifestations of malignancy. Ultimately the patient dies from either major opportunistic infection or malignancy.

   There is no known cure for HIV disease; however, life has been extended in some patients with use of zidovudine (AZT) therapy. Recently the introduction of pentamidine inhaler for prophylactic and therapeutic management of pneumocystis infection has achieved a significant level of success.

3. **Dental therapy:** A single standard for infection control and operator protection should be used when treating all patients. This includes Centers for Disease Control recommendations for barrier technique and ADA recommendations on instrument sterilization and operatory disinfection. For the asymptomatic HIV-positive patient there are no special considerations in rendering dental care. The role of the dentist is to maintain optimum oral health and prevent infectious processes. Often hairy leukoplakia or oral candidiasis may be the first sign of HIV-related disease and can be instrumental in establishing the diagnosis. Recently an AIDS-related peridontitis and gingivitis has been identified, which is rapidly progressive and usually becomes necrotic and purulent. Dental intervention includes management of gingivitis and periodontitis and oral candidiasis, accomplished with mechanical therapy and use of chlorhexidine (Peridex) oral rinses. Many patients with AIDS demonstrate idiopathic thrombocytopenic purpura (ITP), which causes significant depletion of platelets and ultimately presents a bleeding risk. If surgical procedures are considered, bleeding time must be determined, and in consultation with the patient's physician it must be decided whether the patient is an acceptable candidate for oral surgery. As HIV disease progresses into the final stage, the oral health role is primarily palliative, to relieve pain and control infection.

XVII. **CANCER**
   A. **Head and neck radiation therapy**
      1. **Definition/description:** Radiation therapy to the head and neck region can be used as a primary source of treatment, as presurgical treatment to shrink a tumor to more operable size, or after operation to treat surgical margins and prevent recurrence. The usual dose ranges from 5,000 to 7,000 Gy (5,000 to 7,000 rad) delivered over 6 to 7 weeks at approximately 1,500 to 2,000 Gy per treatment.

2. **Signs/symptoms:** Radiation therapy is often successful in shrinking or eradicating tumors, but can be associated with extensive side effects. Radiation affects mucosal tissue, salivary gland tissue, and bone. These effects are manifested by a generalized mucositis, salivary gland dysfunction leading to xerostomia, and major compromise of the intraosseous vasculature. There are also muscle contractures or constrictures and variable loss of taste. Secondary side effects include an increased risk for cervical caries due to xerostomia and for intraoral infections, primarily fungal and viral.

3. **Dental therapy:** All patients scheduled to receive radiation therapy to the head and neck region should undergo an oral health examination. Clinical and radiographic analyses are used to formulate a treatment plan that provides for the removal of all hopelessly periodontally involved or nonrestorable teeth, endodontic treatment of periapical disease, periodontal therapy, and restoration of teeth with minimal caries. At this time the patient is counseled regarding the need for fastidious oral hygiene and the consequences of radiation therapy, including xerostomia, mucositis, and the impact on gingival tissues. Impressions should be made for the fabrication of soft vacuum-formed splints, which will be used to carry flouride gel twice a day. Once this therapy has been accomplished the patient should be cleared for radiation therapy. During radiation therapy the patient should be monitored every 2 to 3 weeks to ensure that oral hygiene is being maintained and to treat symptoms of mucositis. Mucositis has been successfully treated by the use of chlorhexidine (Peridex) rinses. After completion of radiation therapy the patient is seen every 2 to 3 months to ensure that hygiene is being maintained and caries, if they should develop, are treated. It is important to understand that the patient who has received radiation therapy, particularly to the mandible, is at risk for osteoradionecrosis. If 6 months or more after radiation the patient presents in acute

distress, every effort should be made to avoid extraction of teeth; even nonrestorable teeth should be treated endodontically in lieu of extraction. If surgery is required, preparation of the patient with hyperbaric oxygen and antibiotic therapy has been moderately successful in avoiding development of osteoradionecrosis.

B. Chemotherapy

1. **Definition/description:** Cancer chemotherapy involves infusion of cytotoxic pharmacologic agents directed at tumor cells. There are many side effects and complications to normal healthy cells. Chemotherapy may be the sole form of treatment for a particular tumor or used in conjunction with surgical treatment or radiation therapy.

2. **Clinical presentation/symptoms:** The major side effects of cancer chemotherapy and preparation for bone marrow transplantation are due to bone marrow suppression. Thrombocytopenia, leukopenia, or anemia may result from therapy. Oral and intestinal mucosa is also affected, with resultant mucositis, and gastric distress and diarrhea. The severity and duration of side effects vary with the type of therapeutic agent and protocol used.

3. **Dental therapy:** All patients prepared for chemotherapy or bone marrow transplantation should receive dental consultation. At that time clinical and radiographic evaluation is performed and a treatment plan designed. These patients are at significant risk for infection. Teeth with even a marginal prognosis should be removed before therapy. At the same time, complete prophylaxis and periodontal therapy should be performed, as well as caries control. Patients are counseled regarding the need for fastidious oral hygiene and are made aware of anticipated mucosal and gingival changes. Mechanical home care should be modified during therapy. As marrow suppression occurs, tissue may become friable and subject to bleeding and ulceration on mechanical debridement. Home care should consist of using soft gauze or other material for gentle debride-

ment and the use of chlorhexidine rinse to help alleviate the pain and discomfort of mucositis, reduce plaque formation, and maintain gingival tone. Patients should be monitored regularly during chemotherapy to assess the amount of soft tissue involvement, including viral or fungal lesions. If herpetic lesions are discovered, an aggressive treatment plan of acyclovir (Zovirax) should be initiated in conjunction with the patient's oncologist. Fungal lesions can be managed topically with chlorhexidine, nystatin (Mycostatin), or clotrimazole (Mycelex) or systemically with ketoconazole (Nizoral). If acute episodes develop during therapy, consultation with the oncologist must be sought immediately. If invasive procedures are contemplated, great care must be taken if the patient's white blood cell count is less than 1,000 cells/mm^3 or if platelet count is below 40,000/mm^3. Antibiotics and analgesics can be used palliatively until definitive care can be rendered. This may involve hospitalization, with transfusion of platelets and other hematologic support. If possible palliatively therapy should be sustained until a window between therapeutic sessions is found. When surgical care is rendered, antibiotic prophylaxis should be used for infection control, with aggressive local measures to control bleeding.

XVIII. BLEEDING DISORDERS

A. Platelet dysfunction

1. **Definition/description:** Thrombocytopenia, a decrease in platelet number, can lead to bleeding episodes. Many thrombocytopenias are drug-induced, particularly by thiazide diuretics, methyldopa, and quinine. Immune thrombocytopenic purpura is rapid platelet destruction caused by an immune mediated response. Episodes may be acute or chronic. Myeloproliferative disorders can also cause bone marrow suppression and decreased platelet function. Finally, hypersplenism may cause sequestration of platelets.

   Another form of platelet disorders involves acquired or congenital platelet dysfunction. von

Willebrand's disease is a congenital platelet disorder characterized by a deficiency in the synthesis of a plasma factor necessary for platelet function as well as decrease of factor VIII. Platelet function can be impaired by aspirin use, which can diminish platelet function for 7 to 10 days. Nonsteroidal anti-inflammatory drugs have a negative effect on platelet function, which lasts up to 6 hours. Patients with uremia have bleeding disorders secondary to platelet dysfunction.

2. **Clinical presentation/symptoms:** The most common presentation of platelet dysfunction is petechial lesions on either the skin or the mucosa. A platelet count will establish the number of platelets present, and bleeding time will assess platelet function.

B. **Coagulopathies**

1. **Definition/description:** Hemophilia A is a congenital disorder due to factor VIII deficiency. Severity of the disease varies with the level of factor: less than 1% factor is considered severe hemophilia, 1% to 5% factor is considered moderate hemophilia, and 6% to 30% factor is considered mild hemophilia. Hemophilia B is factor IX deficiency, with much lower frequency in the population than hemophilia A. Both are inherited in a sex-linked recessive mode.

Coagulopathies can also be acquired as a result of liver disease or malabsorption syndromes. Inasmuch as the liver is responsible for synthesis of many coagulation factors, hepatic failure or alcoholic cirrhosis can severely compromise coagulation ability. In a malabsorption state there is an inability to absorb vitamin K; therefore vitamin K–dependent coagulation factors cannot be manufactured.

Patients at risk for thromboembolism may be given oral anticoagulants, particularly warfarin sodium (Coumadin), which prevents synthesis of vitamin K–dependent factors. Within a hospital setting patients may be given parenteral heparin therapy. Heparin has a rapid onset of action, with half-life approximately 4 to 6 hours. The presence of a co-agulopathy may become apparent to the patient because of an episode of spontaneous bleeding. More commonly, a patient will experience a bleeding problem after a surgical procedure. These episodes will precipitate further investigation. On normal presurgical screening, abnormalities in prothrombin time (PT), partial thromboplastin time (PTT), or platelet count may be apparent.

2. **Dental therapy:** The potential for bleeding episodes should be of concern to all clinicians. A history of spontaneous bleeding or extensive bleeding after a procedure requires further investigation. Evidence of bleeding disorders in the family should cause concern. A history that provides information concerning the use of particular drugs that induce bleeding should be elicited to evaluate their effect on therapy. Four tests are available that can give important information about the bleeding profile: (1) Platelet count provides the number of platelets. Normal count is 100,000 to 400,000/mm^3. Thrombocytopenia is considered present if platelet count is less than 50,000/mm^3. (2) Bleeding time is used to evaluate platelet function. A standard skin stab produces blood for determining whether bleeding time is normal (between 5 and 10 minutes). (3) Prothrombin time reflects the activity of the extrinsic clotting pathway. It is particularly useful in monitoring warfarin therapy, which most cardiologists use to control PT at one and one-half to two times control value. Normal is the control value plus one to one and one-half times that value. (4) Partial thromboplastin time reflects the activity of the intrinsic pathway. The normal range is 25 to 40 seconds. PTT elevated to 5 to 10 seconds above the norm may produce mild bleeding episodes; with PTT above 10 seconds there is risk for significant bleeding episodes.

For the patient with hemophilia A, hemophilia B, or von Willebrand's disease, regular dental care should be encouraged. Dental prophylaxis and scaling may cause slight oozing, and plasma products are rarely needed. Patients can receive comprehensive restorative dental care; however, mandibular block anesthesia should be avoided because of risk of piercing a vessel, with hematoma production that may disseminate into the neck and compress the trachea. Infiltration and intraligamental injections can be used. For tooth extractions, consultation with the hematologist should determine the amount of plasma products or desmopressin needed to raise the factor level to 20 to 50 U/dL. Patients with von Willebrand's disease receive cryoprecipitate, plasma, or desmopressin regardless of baseline factor level. Antifibrinolytic drugs such as 6-aminocaproic acid (Amicar) are given on the day of surgery and for 10 days afterward to prevent clot breakdown. Aggressive local measures including packing and suturing of the site should be used. The patient should be monitored daily over the next 72 hours, the period of greatest risk for clot breakdown.

Major surgical procedures should be done in a hospital with a laboratory experienced in clotting factor assay, and in consultation with a hematologist experienced in hemophilia management.

BIBLIOGRAPHY

Bender IB, Barkan MJ: Dental bacteremia and its relationship to bacterial endocarditis: Preventive measures. *Compend Contin Ed Dent* 1989; 10:472–481.

Bender IB, Naidorf IJ, Garvey GJ: Bacterial endocarditis: A consideration for physician and dentist. *JADA* 1984; 109:415–420.

Council on Community Health, Hospital, Institutional and Medical Affairs, American Dental Association: Guidelines for dental management of patients with cardiovascular disease (draft), Sept 1987.

Dajani AS, et al: Prevention of bacterial endocarditis: Recommendations of the American Heart Association. *JAMA* 1990; 264:2919–2922.

Jacobson JJ, Schweitzer S, DePorter DJ, et al: Chemoprophylaxis of dental patients with prosthetic joints: A simulation model. *J Dent Ed* 1988; 52:599–603.

Lipton R: *Management of Hereditary Clotting Factor Disorders*. Manual of the Comprehensive Hemophilia Treatment Center, Long Island Jewish Medical Center.

Little JW, Falace DA: *Dental Management of the Medically Compromised Patient*, ed 3. St Louis, CV Mosby Co, 1988.

Robertson PB, Greenspan JS (eds): *Perspectives on the Oral Manifestation of AIDS*. Littleton, Mass, PSG Publishing Co, 1988.

Rose LF, Kaye D (eds): *Internal Medicine for Dentistry* ed 2. St Louis, CV Mosby Co, 1990.

Sonis ST, Fazio RC, Fang L: *Principles and Practice of Oral Medicine*. Philadelphia, WB Saunders Co, 1984.

Wintrobe MM, Thorn GW, Adams RD, et al (eds): *Harrison's Principles of Internal Medicine*, ed 7. New York, McGraw-Hill Book Co, 1974.

Chapter 5 _____

Nonodontogenic Lesions of the Oral Cavity and Salivary Glands

Gerard F. Koorbusch

_____

This chapter discusses the clinical features, radiographic findings, pertinent laboratory parameters, and treatment of nonodontogenic lesions of the oral cavity and salivary glands. This diverse group of clinicopathologic entities is subdivided rather arbitrarily into lesions of soft tissue, lesions of bone, and lesions of the salivary glands. Soft tissue lesions are further classified as inflammatory and reactive, benign soft tissue tumors, congenital lesions, and malignant soft tissue tumors; bony lesions are subdivided into benign and malignant categories, because of the extreme diversity of the lesions described; and salivary gland lesions are categorized as obstructive, autoimmune, inflammatory, and neoplastic.

These clinicopathologic entities are discussed using the following format:

1. **Chief complaint:** symptom most frequently reported by the patient with a given lesion, or if the lesion is not symptomatic, the most common clinical finding noted by the dentist.
2. **Clinical features:** major clinical findings, signs, and symptoms typical of the lesion under discussion.
3. **Radiographic features:** most common presentation of the lesion on radiographic examination.
4. **Laboratory findings:** laboratory tests that are useful in establishing the clinical differential diagnosis.
5. **Treatment:** common, effective treatment methods available.

   The histopathology of each lesion is not described, although it is on the basis of histologic findings that the definitive diagnosis of the lesion is made. The treating clinician should obtain a biopsy specimen for pathologic diagnosis prior to initiating definitive therapy for any lesion. When a histologic diagnosis is available, the clinician can be assured that the treatment plan will be appropriate and effective.

I. **NONODONTOGENIC SOFT TISSUE LESIONS**
   A. **Reactive or inflammatory lesions**
      1. **Peripheral giant cell granuloma**
         a. **Chief complaint:** Red to purple mass on the gingiva or alveolar mucosa.
         b. **Clinical features:** The peripheral giant cell granuloma has an etiologic association with trauma (e.g., tooth extraction or denture irritation) and may have a varied clinical appearance. The lesion is more often seen in female patients than in male patients (2:1). This lesion frequently presents as a gingival mass of limited size (usually <2 cm), anterior to the molar regions of the

jaws. The surface may be smooth or granular, and ulceration is common. The lesion is typically red to purple, and is firm to palpation. It appears with slightly greater frequency in the mandible than in the maxilla. The lesion does have the potential to erode the underlying bone.

  c. **Radiographic features:** The radiographic appearance of peripheral giant cell granuloma is most frequently within the range of normal; however, bone underlying the lesion may be eroded and appear as an irregular radiolucency.

  d. **Treatment:** Surgical excision of peripheral giant cell granuloma including osteoplasty of the underlying bone in the edentulous jaw should minimize the potential for recurrence of this lesion. Attention should also be directed at removal of any local factors that could act as irritants and stimulate recurrence.

2. **Pyogenic granuloma**

  a. **Chief complaint:** Red, friable mass anywhere on the oral mucosa, but most especially on the attached gingiva.

  b. **Clinical features:** Pyogenic granuloma is a rapidly developing, often painless mass on the mucosa, which may bleed easily if traumatized. The lesion occurs predominantly on the gingiva as a soft, red to purple, compressible mass. Other intraoral sites include the lips, tongue, and buccal mucosa. Microtrauma is thought to cause this lesion. Pyogenic granulomas are also called "pregnancy tumors," because they tend to occur commonly in the third month of pregnancy or later and usually regress after delivery. The lesion shows a predilection for occurrence in female patients, and is most often seen in adolescents and young adults. The surface of the lesion may be smooth or ulcerated, and the base may be sessile or pedunculated. These lesions may reach substantial size if left untreated.

  c. **Treatment:** Surgical excision is the treatment of

choice for pyogenic granuloma. The adjacent
teeth should be scaled at the time of surgery to
reduce irritation during healing and reduce the
potential for recurrence. In the pregnant patient a
greater success rate with primary excision may
be achieved if surgery is delayed until after delivery, if possible.

3. **Fibroma**
   a. **Chief complaint:** Painless mass on the lips, buc-
      cal mucosa, gingiva, tongue, or palate.
   b. **Clinical features:** The fibroma is a slow-
      growing benign lesion frequently associated with
      a history of trauma, such as a cheek bite or from
      ill-fitting dentures. The mass may be soft or firm
      to palpation, and is usually of normal color. The
      surface of the lesion may be smooth or ulcerated;
      the base may be sessile or pedunculated. The
      lesion is typically small; however, fibromas of
      long duration may enlarge to several centimeters
      in diameter if left untreated. There is no gender
      or age predilection for these lesions.
   c. **Treatment:** Simple surgical excision is the treat-
      ment of choice for fibroma; recurrence is un-
      likely.

4. **Traumatic neuroma**
   a. **Chief complaint:** Small nodular swelling.
   b. **Clinical features:** Traumatic neuroma is a non-
      neoplastic exuberant attempt of the body to re-
      pair a damaged nerve. The lesion is common at
      the site of previous surgery or trauma. It is usu-
      ally discrete, less than 1 cm in diameter, nodu-
      lar, tender, and often found in the region of the
      mental foramen. Pressure applied to the lesion
      usually causes pain in the region or throughout
      the distribution of the nerve.
   c. **Treatment:** Surgical excision of traumatic neu-
      roma should be curative; however, nerve resec-
      tion may induce formation of a secondary neu-
      roma. Microsurgical resection may be appropri-
      ate to preserve sensation and minimize neural
      trauma in selected cases.

B. Benign soft tissue tumors

1. Peripheral ossifying fibroma

a. **Chief complaint:** Gingival mass.

b. **Clinical features:** This lesion often arises as a discrete mass within the interdental papilla. It is found in children and young adults, and is more common in female patients. The maxillary and mandibular arches are affected with equal frequency. The anterior portions of the dentoalveolar ridge (anterior to the molar teeth) is the most common site of occurrence. The mass may be sessile or pedunculated. The mucosa may be intact or ulcerated.

c. **Radiographic features:** In most patients, radiographs of the area of the lesion are unremarkable. However, in some patients erosion of bone may be noted beneath the lesion.

d. **Treatment:** Surgical excision of these benign soft tissue tumors is the treatment of choice. Histologic diagnosis is mandatory, because the recurrence rate for this lesion is 15% to 20%.

2. Keratoacanthoma

a. **Chief complaint:** Mass on the lower lip.

b. **Clinical features:** This benign lesion most often presents as a rapidly growing mass of the lip, reaching maximum size in 1 to 2 months. The keratoacanthoma clinically appears as an elevated crater with a central core of keratin and rolled borders. The lesion is usually less than 2 cm in diameter, and may undergo spontaneous regression with time. The lesion may be painful, with associated regional lymphadenopathy. The overall clinical appearance of the lesion is consistent with carcinoma of the lip, although the lesion is benign. The keratoacanthoma is a focal form of pseudoepitheliomatous hyperplasia. It is seen twice as frequently in males than in female patients, and most often affects persons between 50 and 70 years of age.

c. **Treatment:** Surgical excision of keratoacanthoma is required because of its suspect clinical appearance. The diagnosis of keratoacanthoma can be made only on the basis of histologic findings, not clinical findings. In addition, spontaneous regression does not always occur; thus surgical excision remains the indicated treatment. Recurrence after excision is rare.

3. **Granular cell myoblastoma**
   a. **Chief complaint:** Mass in the tongue.
   b. **Clinical features:** This lesion occurs approximately 50% of the time in the substance of the tongue. It is usually a solitary nodule found along the lateral border or dorsum of the tongue. The overlying mucosa is commonly normal, but may have a whitish hue. The lesion is painless, soft to palpation, and slow growing. There is no apparent gender or age predilection.
   c. **Treatment:** Simple surgical excision is the treatment of choice for granular cell myoblastoma, and there is little likelihood of recurrence.

4. **Papilloma**
   a. **Chief complaint:** Well-circumscribed mass of the oral cavity, with a wartlike surface and appearance.
   b. **Clinical features:** Papilloma is slow growing up to a certain size, after which growth appears to arrest. The lesion is common in the oral cavity. It can occur at any age, but is seen most frequently between 20 and 50 years of age. The lesion occurs on the lips, buccal mucosa, tongue, and palate (especially near the uvula). The surface appears cauliflower-like, with a pedunculated or less frequently sessile base. Multiple lesions have been reported in individual patients. A viral agent, human papillomavirus, has been detected in at least some oral squamous papillomas.
   c. **Treatment:** Simple surgical excision of the papilloma including its base is the treatment of choice, with little likelihood of recurrence.

5. **Neurolemmoma (schwannoma)**
   a. **Chief complaint:** Soft tissue mass of the oral cavity.

   b. **Clinical features:** Neurolemmoma is a tumor of nerve sheath origin that is slow growing and often chronic. The tumor most commonly occurs in the head and neck, and the lesion may apply pressure to surrounding or adjacent neural tissue, with resulting pain or numbness in these areas. The most common intraoral sites are the palate, floor of the mouth, buccal mucosa, and gingiva. The lesions are encapsulated. Intraosseous lesions have been reported, with the mandible affected more frequently than the maxilla. Central lesions often produce expansion of bony cortical plates and associated pain and paresthesia.
   c. **Radiographic features:** Central lesions appear as delinated and expansile radiolucencies.
   d. **Treatment:** The treatment of neurolemmoma is surgical excision. Because the tumor is encapsulated, surgical excision is usually curative, and recurrence is rare.
6. **Neurofibroma**
   a. **Chief complaint:** Solitary or multiple soft tissue lesion of the oral cavity.
   b. **Clinical features:** The neurofibroma, caused by proliferation of Schwann cells, occurs without gender or racial predilection. The lesion is a slow-growing, solitary, multiple or disseminated mass and can occur anywhere in the oral cavity. The disseminated form, von Recklinghausen's disease, is inherited as an autosomal dominant trait with variable penetrance, and is characterized by diffuse neurofibromatosis, café-au-lait spots, and potential malignant degeneration of the tumors.

   Oral neurofibromas are covered by mucosa of normal color and may be distributed throughout the palate, vestibule, buccal mucosa, alveolar ridge, and tongue. Macroglossia is a sequela of diffuse involvement of the tongue. The lesions are not encapsulated. Central lesions have been reported, and are typically found in the mandible in association with the mandibular canal.

c. **Radiographic features:** Central lesions appear as diffuse radiolucent enlargements of the mandibular canal, often producing "blunderbuss" expansion of the inferior alveolar foramen.

d. **Treatment:** Solitary neurofibromas may be excised without significant incidence of recurrence. Neurofibromatosis has no specific treatment; thus surgical therapy is primarily for cosmetic or functional purposes only.

7. **Lipoma**
   a. **Chief complaint:** Painless yellowish submucosal mass in the oral cavity.
   b. **Clinical features:** The lipoma is a slow-growing, painless tumor of mature fat cells. The neoplasm occurs infrequently in the oral cavity. It is primarily seen in adult patients as a yellowish mass with thin overlying mucosa. The lesion may occur as a nodular or lobulated mass on a sessile or pedunculated base. The most common sites of occurrence in the oral cavity are the tongue, floor of the mouth, and buccal mucosa. The lipoma is minimally encapsulated and typically soft to palpation.
   c. **Treatment:** Lipoma requires simple surgical excision; there is little likelihood of recurrence.

8. **Leiomyoma**
   a. **Chief complaint:** Painless soft tissue mass in the oral cavity.
   b. **Clinical features:** Leiomyoma, an uncommon tumor of the mouth, most often presents as a slow-growing, painless mass. It is a tumor of smooth muscle, seen more frequently in females than in males, and in middle-aged patients. The most frequent site of occurrence is on the posterior aspects of the tongue, but can develop virtually anywhere in the oral cavity. The lesion is typically encapsulated and firm, but may be multinodular.
   c. **Treatment:** Leiomyoma is treated by simple surgical excision.

C. Congenital lesions
1. Hemangioma
   a. **Chief complaint:** Red to purple lesion of the head and neck.
   b. **Clinical features:** Hemangioma, the most common tumor of the head and neck in childhood, often is congenital or develops shortly after birth. Hemangioma typically is solitary, and may regress as the patient matures. The lesion is more common in girls than in boys, and appears intraorally as a red or purple mass of the mucosa. The most common sites of occurrence are the lips, tongue, buccal mucosa, and palate. These lesions may become traumatized, ulcerated, or secondarily infected.

   Central hemangioma of the jaw occurs infrequently and often is difficult to diagnose. Central lesions are of varying size and invariably osseodestructive.
   c. **Radiographic features:** Soft tissue hemangioma may undergo phlebolithiasis, that is, formation of calcified stones in the complex facial vascular structure. These phleboliths may appear on facial or oral radiographs as circular or ovoid radiopacities that are well-circumscribed.

   Central lesions appear cystlike or honeycombed.
   d. **Treatment:** Some congenital hemangiomas regress during childhood. Traditional treatments include surgical excision, sclerosing agents, cryotherapy, and embolization. Radiation therapy is no longer considered an acceptable form of therapy.

Diagnosis of hemangioma may require angiography prior to structuring a definitive treatment plan. Because suspected central vascular lesions have the potential for substantial hemorrhage during surgical exploration, preoperative aspiration should be performed to ensure that this life-threatening complication is avoided. If the aspirate contains blood, surgical intervention should be deferred until definitive angiography is performed.

Definitive care of vascular lesions should be performed only by qualified surgeons in the controlled environment of a hospital operating room.

   2. **Lymphangioma**
      a. **Chief complaint:** Congenital soft tissue enlarge-ment of the oral cavity.
      b. **Clinical features:** Lymphangioma is a malfor-mation or hamartoma of the lymphatic vessels. The lesions are noted at birth or shortly thereaf-ter. There is no gender predilection in the occur-rence of the lesion, but the head and neck is in-volved in 50% of the cases. The most common site of occurrence is the tongue. Progressive en-largement of the lesion is associated with macro-glossia and apertognathia. Other sites of expres-sion of this disease include the palate, buccal mucosa, gingiva, and lips. Superficial lesions are often papillary; deeper lesions appear nodular. These lesions may be of normal color or larger lesions of the tongue may appear grey-pink. Le-sions of the lip may cause macrocheilia. The lesions tend to enlarge slowly until puberty, after which growth may cease.
      c. **Treatment:** Surgical excision or revision is the treatment of choice for lymphangioma. Sponta-neous regression of the lesion is rare.
   D. **Malignant soft tissue tumors**
      1. **Fibrosarcoma**
         a. **Chief complaint:** Mass of the face causing asymmetry.
         b. **Clinical features:** Fibrosarcoma is an uncommon tumor of the head and neck. This malignant tu-mor can arise anywhere in the head and neck, but is usually noted in the cheek, sinus, pharynx, lip, and periosteal regions of the jaws, usually before age 50 years. The tumor may be rapid or slow growing, but is invariably invasive locally. The lesion is fleshy and bulky, and may become ulcerated, infected, or bleed spontaneously. Cen-tral forms of the tumor have been reported, and appear radiographically as diffuse osteolytic le-sions.

    c. **Treatment:** Treatment of the fibrosarcoma is via radical surgical excision.

2. **Melanoma**

    a. **Chief complaint:** Pigmented lesion of the oral cavity.

    b. **Clinical features:** This aggressive melanocyte malignancy rarely occurs in the oral cavity. The lesion is most often found in patients of middle age (40 to 70 years), and is more common in male patients. The oral expression of the lesion is more common in Japanese than in other patient groups. The tumor usually presents as a deeply pigmented brown or blue-black mass intraorally. The most common oral site for the tumor is the anterior palate and the maxillary alveolar ridge, often arising in preexisting mucosal melanosis. The lesion may present as a fungating mass or with ulceration and bleeding as well as pigmentation. Nonpigmented forms of the tumor have been reported.

    c. **Treatment:** Radical surgical excision is the primary treatment of melanoma. Regional prophylactic lymph node dissection in patients without frank lymph node involvement is controversial. Adjuvant therapy includes chemotherapy, radiation, and immunotherapy. The long-term prognosis for oral tumors is poor.

3. **Burkitt's lymphoma**

    a. **Chief complaint:** Rapid massive swelling of the jaws.

    b. **Clinical features:** This non-Hodgkin's lymphoma was first discovered in African children, but has subsequently been found in children of various countries, including the United States. The tumor is characterized by massive, very rapid growth, especially in the jaws. The primary areas of expression of the tumor outside of the jaws include the abdominal viscera, lymph nodes, and ovaries. The neoplasm primarily affects children, predominately boys. Facial disfigurement, loose teeth, tooth displacement, and sinus involvement are all clinical facial features of the disease. Patients with Burkitt's lymphoma often have increased titers of antibodies to the Epstein-Barr virus; however, a direct causal relationship has not been established.

c. **Radiographic features:** Burkitt's lymphoma presents with massive destruction of bone. The margins of the lesion are usually indistinct, and the cortices may be expanded, eroded, or perforated.

d. **Treatment:** Burkitt's lymphoma may be controlled with chemotherapy.

4. **Kaposi's sarcoma**
   a. **Chief complaint:** Purple or red-brown lesion of the skin or mucous membrane.
   b. **Clinical features:** Kaposi's sarcoma is a vascular malignancy found on the skin of the lower extremities and the oral cavity. This tumor is seen predominately in male patients. Until recently it was seen infrequently in elderly patients; however, with the epidemic of acquired immune deficiency syndrome (AIDS) a much larger number of younger patients has developed the disease. The lesions of Kaposi's sarcoma are red-brown to purple, variable in size, multiple, and usually painful to palpation. Lesions of the skin and mucous membrane of the oral cavity are identical in appearance.
   c. **Treatment:** Surgical excision is difficult if Kaposi's sarcoma is disseminated. Radiation and chemotherapy have been effective in treating the lesions. The long-term mean survival rate for patients with the tumor alone is about 10 years; however, AIDS patients with the tumor have a much poorer survival rate.

5. **Embryonal rhabdomyosarcoma**
   a. **Chief complaint:** Embryonal rhabdomyosarcoma often presents with pain and swelling.
   b. **Clinical features:** Embryonal rhabdomyosarcoma is an uncommon malignancy, occurring predominantly in young patients, in whom it is the most common head and neck sarcoma. The

tumor grows rapidly, with little in the way of clinically useful diagnostic features. It may occur in the orbit, zygoma, palate, mastoid, internal ear, or temporal and cervical regions. Clinical symptoms may include divergence of the eye, difficulty with speech and swallowing, asymmetry of the jaws or facial skeleton, and discharge from the ears. Thorough and complete medical workup is required in addition to biopsy for the diagnosis and staging of this tumor.

c. **Treatment:** The treatment of embryonal rhabdomyosarcoma involves the integration of wide surgical excision, radiation therapy, and chemotherapeutic protocols for the maximum benefit of the patient. This integrated approach offers hope for control of the tumor and long-term survival of these patients. The overall prognosis with multimodal therapy is closely related to the initial presentation. In nonorbital or meningeal sites the disease-free survival rate is 75%, but falls to 18% with metastatic disease.

6. **Verrucous carcinoma**
   a. **Chief complaint:** Slow-growing white fungating lesion, usually on the mucobuccal fold or the alveolar ridge.
   b. **Clinical features:** Verrucous carcinoma is a slow-growing, low-grade malignancy of the oral cavity, and is noted primarily in older patients who have a history of using snuff or chewing tobacco. Men are affected more frequently than women. The lesion is often white, with an irregular corrugated or folded surface sometimes described as "shaggy." The lesion is found in the mucobuccal fold, alveolar ridge, or buccal mucosa. Verrucous carcinoma tends to spread laterally, with superficial invasion. Potential for metastasis is very low until late in the course of the disease.
   c. **Treatment:** Surgical excision is the treatment of choice for verrucous carcinoma. Radiation is contraindicated because of the potential for trans-

formation of the lesion into a more anaplastic form, although more recently this concept has been challenged, with good results reported with nonsurgical therapy.

7. **Squamous cell carcinoma**
   a. **Chief complaint:** Painless mass or ulcer of the oral mucosa.
   b. **Clinical features:** Squamous cell carcinoma is the most common oral malignancy. It has been associated with a variety of predisposing factors, including the use of tobacco and alcohol, syphilis, and Plummer-Vinson syndrome. In addition, carcinoma of the lip has been associated with prolonged exposure to the sun.

   The disease is most prevalent in patients older than 40 years, with a distinct male predominance, although in recent studies a growing percentage of cases are in female patients. The lesions may appear as leukoplakias, speckled leukoplakias, or erythroplakias. Common presentations of the tumor include ulcers, exophytic fungating masses, white plaques, and red patches, all of which may be associated with induration and fixation. Cervical lymphadenopathy is frequently associated with oral carcinoma. Intraoral areas that should be considered highly susceptible to oral carcinomatosis include the lateral and ventral surfaces of the tongue, the anterior floor of the mouth, and the tonsillar pillars.

   Ulceration in association with oral carcinoma may appear, with rolled borders and induration, especially on the tongue or lip. Because of the potentially diverse presentation of oral carcinoma, white, red, or speckled lesions of the oral cavity should be biopsied, particularly in patients with any predisposing factors. Any lesion of the type described associated with induration or fixation should be assumed malignant until histopathologic diagnosis proves otherwise.
   c. **Treatment:** Depending on the location and ex-

tent of the tumor, wide surgical excision, regional lymph node dissection, and radiation therapy have been the mainstays of conventional therapy. Specific treatment planning is determined by clinical staging of the tumors and placing such staged tumors into established treatment protocols. Tumor staging is described in Chapter 9.

II. NONODONTOGENIC DISEASES OF BONE
A. Benign conditions of bone
1. Central giant cell granuloma
a. **Chief complaint:** Enlargement of the jaw.

b. **Clinical features:** Central giant cell granuloma is a painless, generally asymptomatic, and slow-growing enlargement of the affected portion of the jaw, most commonly the mandible. The tumor may be discovered incidentally on routine radiographic survey. It is more frequently seen in male patients, typically younger than 30 years of age, and most often anterior to the premolar teeth. The clinical appearance is usually one of normal mucosa overlying an area of buccal or lingual cortical expansion. Root divergence or resorption may be evident.

c. **Radiographic features:** Central giant cell granuloma is seen as a radiolucent lesion with smooth or irregular borders, and may be multilocular.

d. **Laboratory studies:** Evaluation should include laboratory tests for hyperparathyroidism, including serum calcium, phosphorus, and alkaline phosphatase values. In hyperparathyroidism, serum calcium and alkaline phosphatase levels are elevated and serum phosphorus is depressed. No laboratory abnormalities are noted in a patient with central giant cell granuloma without hyperparathyroidism.

e. **Treatment:** The treatment of central giant cell granuloma is local, with thorough curettage and peripheral ostectomy. The anticipated recurrence rate is low.

2. **Ossifying fibroma**
   a. **Chief complaint:** Localized hard swelling or mass in the jaws.
   b. **Clinical features:** This central lesion presents as a slow-growing asymptomatic mass. Ossifying fibroma occurs most frequently in young adults, and shows a marked predilection for the mandible. Female patients are affected more frequently than male patients. The lesion may cause displacement of teeth. A so-called juvenile active form has been described, with a more aggressive presentation.
   c. **Radiographic features:** Ossifying fibroma appears radiolucent in its early stages of growth, but becomes more radiopaque centrally as it matures. Thus the more mature tumors will appear as mixed radiolucent-radiopaque lesions. The lesions appear well demarcated on radiographs, with tooth displacement noted in large lesions in tooth-bearing areas.
   d. **Treatment:** Surgical excision is the treatment of choice for ossifying fibroma. Recurrence of the routine lesion is rare. Aggressive juvenile and diffuse maxillary lesions may require surgical resection if definitive treatment is to be curative.

3. **Osteoid osteoma**
   a. **Chief complaint:** Pain in a localized region of the jaw.
   b. **Clinical features:** Osteoid osteoma is a benign tumor of bone found in young patients, usually before age 30 years. The lesion is uncharacteristically painful for its small size and benign nature, and classically the discomfort is relieved by aspirin. The lesion is seen twice as often in male patients than in female patients. The soft tissue overlying the lesion may be inflamed, tender, and swollen.
   c. **Radiographic features:** Osteoid osteoma appears as a central radiolucency surrounded by a sclerotic rim of bone. The lesion is typically

less than 1 cm in diameter. Some calcification may be noted in the central area of radiolucency.

d. **Treatment:** Surgical excision is usually curative, and recurrence of the lesion is unlikely.

4. **Benign osteoblastoma**
   a. **Chief complaint:** Mass of the jaws.
   b. **Clinical features:** Benign osteoblastoma is an uncommon tumor of the jaws, characterized by rapid expansion, pain, and swelling. The lesion is more frequently encountered in the long bones and vertebrae. The tumor is significant in that it may be misdiagnosed as malignant. The lesion occurs with greatest frequency before age 30 years, with a predilection for males. Histologically the lesion appears related to osteoid osteoma but exceeds 1 cm in diameter. The tumor occurs with equal frequency in the maxilla and the mandible. The teeth adjacent to the tumor may be displaced, and their roots resorbed.
   c. **Radiographic features:** Benign osteoblastoma may appear radiolucent or as a mixed radiolucent mass with radiopaque calcifications centrally. The tumor is usually well circumscribed.
   d. **Treatment:** Surgical excision is the treatment of choice for benign osteoblastoma. En bloc resection should be considered if the lesion recurs.

5. **Fibrous dysplasia**
   a. **Chief complaint:** Firm, asymmetric, slow-growing swelling of the jaws.
   b. **Clinical features:** This idiopathic osseous disease is insidious in onset, and presents as an expansile lesion of bone. Fibrous dysplasia occurs in monostotic solitary and polyostotic disseminated forms. The polyostotic form of the disease (Albright's syndrome) may have a severe expression, with multiple osseous lesions, café-au-lait spots, and endocrine disturbances.
      Fibrous dysplasia becomes clinically evi-

dent in the first two decades of life as a progressive expansion of bone that often causes asymmetry or gross deformity. Facial bone involvement is more common in the maxilla than the mandible. Teeth affected by the lesion may be displaced or tipped by the expanding lesion. Growth of the lesion may accelerate during puberty and pregnancy. The expansion rate of the lesion usually decreases when the skeleton reaches maturity in the third decade of life. The mucosa overlying the lesions of fibrous dysplasia is usually intact.

Clinically the lesions of fibrous dysplasia present as firm bony expansions of the jaws that may cause alterations in occlusion and malformation of the alveolar processes. The lesions may be severely disfiguring, especially when they occur in the maxilla. Surgical eradication may be difficult if the disease process is extensive.

Malignant degeneration in areas of fibrous dysplasia is rare, but has been reported. Such malignant change has been associated with irradiation of the affected areas of bone.

c. **Radiographic features:** Ground glass radiopaque appearance with indistinct margins.

d. **Laboratory findings:** Serum calcium, phosphorus, and alkaline phosphatase levels usually are within normal limits. In young patients, however, serum alkaline phosphatase levels frequently are elevated, because growth is associated with elevations of this parameter.

e. **Treatment:** Fibrous dysplasia should be treated when there is functional impairment or significant facial deformity. Whenever possible, surgical intervention should be delayed until skeletal maturity has been achieved, at which time the lesions often become quiescent. Because there is the potential, albeit rare, for malignant degeneration of these lesions, long-term follow-up is mandatory. Exacerbation of growth in a quiescent lesion in an adult patient should cause suspicion of malignant change. Such lesions should be biopsied and pathologically evaluated.

6. **Osteoma**
   a. **Chief complaint:** Painless, bony hard mass of the jaws.
   b. **Clinical features:** Osteoma is an uncommon lesion of the jaws that has the potential to cause facial asymmetry. The lesion is a slow-growing, bony hard mass that results from osseous proliferation in the periosteum or endosteum. Osteoma is most often seen in young adults. Osteomas are usually asymptomatic and thus may be discovered incidentally during routine examination.

   Of particular significance is the association of facial bone osteomas with **Gardner's syndrome,** which consists of (1) multiple osteomas of facial bones, (2) epidermoid cysts of skin, (3) intestinal polyposis with a high potential for malignant degeneration, (4) desmoids or fibromas of skin, and (5) multiple impacted or supernumerary teeth.

   The significance of Gardner's syndrome is the potential for development of malignancies of the bowel early in the course of the disease; thus timely recognition of this syndrome is essential for effective treatment.
   c. **Radiographic features:** Well-circumscribed radiopaque mass.
   d. **Treatment:** Osteomas that are chronically irritated or prevent prosthodontic reconstruction of the dental arches should be removed. Simple surgical excision using rotary instruments or osteotomes is usually followed by an uneventful course, and recurrence is rare.

7. **Cherubism**
   a. **Chief complaint:** Bilateral swelling of the jaws during childhood.
   b. **Clinical features:** Cherubism is an uncommon

autosomal dominant hereditary disease with variable expressivity. Typically the penetrance of the disease is 100% in males and 50% to 70% in females. The disease is usually noted in early childhood, and is characterized by slow, progressive swelling of either or both jaws. The lesions are firm or hard to palpation, and regional lymphadenopathy often is present. The deciduous teeth may exfoliate early, and the permanent teeth may be absent, displaced, or refuse to erupt. The angles of the mandible are the most frequently involved regions of the jaws. A chubby face (compared to the classic description of a cherub) is characteristic.

   c. **Radiographic features:** Extensive radiolucent destruction of one or both jaws is noted, with multiple displaced or unerupted teeth. The lesions are well defined and may be multilocular. Perforation of the cortical plates is possible.

   d. **Laboratory findings:** All laboratory test results should be within the range of normal.

   e. **Treatment:** The jaw lesions regress as the patient approaches puberty. Surgical correction for cosmetic purposes after puberty may be indicated if the deformity creates social or psychologic problems. In adulthood the radiographic appearance of the jaws is usually normal.

8. **Eosinophilic granuloma (histiocytosis X)**
   a. **Chief complaint:** Loose teeth, delayed surgical healing, or chronic oral ulceration.
   b. **Clinical features:** Eosinophilic granuloma is part of the disease triad termed histiocytosis X; also included are Hand-Schüller-Christian disease, and Letterer-Siwe disease. Hand-Schüller-Christian disease is the disseminated chronic form of the disease, usually discovered by age 5 years. It is treatable, with an acceptable prognosis. Letterer-Siwe disease is the acute fulminating form of the disease, typically discovered by age 3 years. The prognosis is poor. Only eosinophilic granuloma is discussed here, be-

cause this is the form of the disease most likely to be encountered by the dentist.

Eosinophilic granuloma is characterized by destruction of bone caused by a proliferation of histiocyte-like cells. The lesion is found in adolescents and young adults. The disease occurs twice as frequently in males as in females. The lesion may be discovered as an incidental finding on a radiograph. The skull and the mandible are common sites for the disease, but the femur, humerus, ribs, and other bones may also be affected. General malaise and fever have been associated with onset of the disease. The lesions are characterized by the replacement of bone with "histiocyte" or Langerhans cell granuloma formation.

   c. **Radiographic features:** The lesions of eosinophilic granuloma are round to ovoid radiolucencies that are well demarcated. The teeth associated with the lesions often appear to be floating in space. The lesions may be consistent with advanced periodontal disease.

   d. **Treatment:** These lesions respond quite favorably to enucleation and curettage. Lesions not amenable to surgical treatment can be eradicated effectively with low-dose radiation therapy. More recently intralesional corticosteroid injection has proved of value.

9. **Hyperparathyroidism**

   a. **Chief complaint:** Pathologic fracture or central osteolytic lesion of the jaws.

   b. **Clinical features:** Hyperparathyroidism occurs in primary and secondary forms. The primary form of the disease is caused by parathyroid adenoma, whereas the secondary form is caused by renal failure or endocrine-secreting carcinomas, such as oat cell carcinoma of the lung. Patients are usually of middle age, and three times as many females than males are affected. Often a pathologic feature or "jaw cyst" is the initiating symptom of the disease. Jaw lesions are brown tumors, which are virtually indistinguishable from the central giant cell granuloma of bone. The lesions may be multiple and bilateral, and may affect multiple areas of the skeleton. It has been estimated that half of all patients with hyperparathyroidism have no symptoms.

c. **Radiographic features:** Generalized radiolucency of the skeleton is noted, with loss of the lamina dura around teeth. As the disease progresses, radiolucent punctate lesions are noted in the maxilla and mandible. These jaw lesions are consistent with the brown tumors of hyperparathyroidism.

d. **Laboratory findings:** Elevation of the serum calcium or serum parathyroid hormone levels. (Of clinical significance is the increased incidence of urinary tract stones, fatigue, depression, mental confusion, anorexia, vomiting, constipation, renal tubular defects, increased urination, and cardiac arrhythmias associated with increased serum calcium levels.)

e. **Treatment:** Primary hyperparathyroidism requires excision of the parathyroid gland(s). Secondary hyperparathyroidism requires treatment of the underlying disease.

10. **Paget's disease**

a. **Chief complaint:** Slow progressive enlargement of the jaws in an elderly patient.

b. **Clinical features:** The cause of Paget's disease is not known. The disease is found predominantly in patients older than 40 years, with a slight predilection for occurrence in male patients. This is a slowly developing chronic disease that causes progressive enlargement of the skull and deformities of the spine, femur, and tibia. The involved bones are warm to the touch due to increased vascularity, and may fracture easily. Bone pain, headache, deafness, blindness, dizziness, facial nerve paralysis, and mental disturbances are related to direct involvement of the cranial foramina. In the jaws the maxilla is involved more frequently than the mandible. In the maxilla, alveolar widening and palatal flattening are noted. Inability to wear dentures is a common complaint in these patients.

The lesions of Paget's disease have a limited tendency to undergo malignant degeneration to osteosarcoma.

c. **Radiographic features:** The characteristic appearance of the lesions of Paget's disease has been described as patchy "cotton-wool" radiopacities of the skull and jaws. Dental radiographs may demonstrate hypercementosis and loss of the lamina dura in affected areas of the jaws. Root resorption has been reported, but is not common.

d. **Laboratory findings:** Serum calcium and phosphorus levels usually are within normal limits; however, the alkaline phosphatase value is extremely high during the osteoblastic phase of the disease.

e. **Treatment:** There is no specific treatment for Paget's disease. Calcitonin has been used for treatment of the active phases of the disease, with inconclusive results.

B. **Malignancies of bone**
 1. **Ewing's sarcoma**
  a. **Chief complaint:** Rapid development of pain and swelling in the jaws.
  b. **Clinical features:** Ewing's sarcoma is an uncommon tumor of bone, which occasionally involves the jaws. The tumor is most common in children and young adults, and there is a definite male predilection. The tumor has been frequently reported to occur after an episode of trauma, but there is no evidence of a causal relationship between the two. The lesion most frequently occurs in the long bones, skull, clavicles, ribs, shoulder, and pelvic girdle. When it occurs in the jaws there seems to be a greater

frequency in the mandible. The lesion presents as a painful swelling of bone, and in the jaws may be associated with facial neuralgia and lip paresthesia. The tumor is also associated with fever and an elevated white blood cell count and thus gives the impression of infection to the clinician. Intraoral masses are rapidly growing and may become ulcerated. Rapid hematogenous metastasis is an early potential sequela of this tumor.

c. **Radiographic findings:** Ewing's sarcoma presents as a destructive diffuse radiolucent mass, with the formation of subperiosteal bone in a layered pattern. This onion skin appearance is classic for the tumor; however, it is also possible for the tumor to appear with osteophyte formation and give the "sunray" appearance often associated with osteosarcoma.

d. **Laboratory findings:** Leukocytosis is frequently encountered in patients with Ewing's sarcoma.

e. **Treatment:** Treatment of Ewing's sarcoma is with combined surgery, radiation therapy, and chemotherapy. Traditionally, survival rates for patients with this tumor have been poor.

2. **Multiple myeloma**
   a. **Chief complaint:** Pain and swelling in the jaw.
   b. **Clinical features:** Multiple myeloma is a disseminated malignant disease of cells of bone marrow origin. The disease mainly affects patients between 40 and 70 years of age, with males more frequently affected than females. The predominant clinical feature of the disease is pain, and pathologic fracture commonly is encountered during the course of the disease. In the jaws the mandible is the site of the disease in the vast majority of the patients. Oral symptoms include pain, swelling, jaw expansion, paresthesia, tooth mobility, extraosseous gingival lesions, and spread to the lymph nodes, skin, and viscera.

c. **Radiographic features:** Numerous punched out radiolucencies of the vertebrae, skull, ribs, jaws, and long bones are noted. These lesions are found with the greatest frequency in areas of active hematopoietic activity. Infrequently an osteoblastic form of the disease may occur.

d. **Laboratory findings:** Anemia, hypercalcemia, hyperglobulinemia, reversal of the albumin-globulin ratio, increased total protein, and urinary Bence-Jones proteins may be associated with multiple myeloma.

e. **Treatment:** Treatment is directed at control of this disseminated disease through the use of chemotherapy. Radiation may be used palliatively to control specific areas of osseous involvement.

3. **Osteosarcoma (osteogenic sarcoma)**

   a. **Chief complaint:** Mass of the jaws associated with rapid growth and pain.

   b. **Clinical features:** This malignant tumor is rare in the jaws, but is most commonly encountered in long bones, especially the femur and tibia. The tumor shows a predilection for young patients, 10 to 25 years old, and occurs with greater frequency in males. The lesion is generally described in terms of two types: the osteolytic form (less well differentiated) and the osteoblastic or sclerosing form. This neoplasm has been associated with occurrence or discovery after some traumatic episode. There is definitely a higher incidence of the tumor in patients with Paget's disease and in those who have received radiation to the area of the tumor.

   In the jaws, osteosarcoma typically appears as a painful mass. The tumor is more common in the mandible, in males, and in patients approximately a decade older than those in which the tumor occurs in long bones. Common symptoms associated with osteosarcoma in the jaw include pain, paresthesia, facial deformity, loose teeth, bleeding, odontalgia, and nasal obstruction.

c. **Radiographic features:** The earliest sign of osteosarcoma of the jaws is localized symmetric widening of the periodontal ligament. This sign is seen only in this tumor, scleroderma, and acrosclerosis, and thus is a significant radiographic feature. In the osteoblastic (sclerosing) variety the typical sunray appearance may be noted radiographically on the periphery of the lesion. The osteolytic form of the tumor does not have distinctive radiographic features, and may appear as a destructive irregular radiolucency of the jaws.

d. **Treatment:** Radical surgical excision with adjuvant chemotherapy is the treatment of choice for osteosarcoma. Complete surgical excision of these tumors may be difficult in the head and neck, because of the close proximity or invasion of vital structures.

III. DISORDERS OF SALIVARY GLANDS
A. Obstructive lesions
1. Mucocele

a. **Chief complaint:** Fluctuant mass of the lower lip.

b. **Clinical features:** A cystlike lesion of the minor salivary glands, the mucocele is found on the lower lip in greater than 90% of cases, as well as on the buccal mucosa and the ventral surface of the tongue. These very common lesions are susceptible to trauma and may rupture spontaneously. They arise rapidly, are usually painless, fluctuant, and are blue or red. The mucocele is thought to arise via the extravasation of saliva into the tissues secondary to the traumatic severance of a minor salivary gland duct or by obstruction of a salivary gland duct.

c. **Treatment:** Surgical excision is the treatment of choice, with special attention to removal of the underlying minor salivary gland lobule to minimize the potential for recurrence.

   2. **Ranula**
      a. **Chief complaint:** Fluctuant swelling of the
         floor of the mouth.
      b. **Clinical features:** Ranula is best described as a
         mucocele of the floor of the mouth secondary to
         extravasation of the sublingual gland saliva into
         the surrounding soft tissue. The lesion is usu-
         ally painless, and may cause deviation of the
         tongue as it enlarges. It may less commonly
         arise as a submental or submandibular mass,
         called a plunging ranula.
      c. **Treatment:** Surgical excision or marsupializa-
         tion (unroofing) is the recommended treatment
         for ranula. Recurrence or very large size may
         mandate surgical removal of the sublingual
         gland.
B. **Autoimmune disorders**
   1. **Sjögren's syndrome**
      a. **Chief complaint:** Swelling of the parotid
         glands, dry eyes, dry mouth, and associated
         connective tissue disease.
      b. **Clinical features:** Sjögren's syndrome classi-
         cally is described as consisting of keratocon-
         junctivitis sicca, xerostomia, and rheumatoid
         arthritis. The disease affects primarily the mid-
         dle aged, and shows a marked (10:1) predilec-
         tion for female patients. The disease is immu-
         nologic, and may be associated with lymphade-
         nopathy, purpura, Raynaud's phenomenon, kid-
         ney involvement, and myositis. Symptoms
         include dryness of the eyes and mouth and a
         burning sensation of the oral mucosa. Patients
         with Sjögren's syndrome have an increased risk
         for lymphoma.
      c. **Radiographic features:** Sialography of the pa-
         rotid glands will demonstrate sialectasia, with
         punctate defects filled with radiopaque dye in
         the "cherry blossom" pattern.
      d. **Laboratory findings:** The patient may have an
         elevated erythrocyte sedimentation rate, positive
         rheumatoid factor, positive antinuclear antibod-

ies, and decreased tearing as determined by Schirmer test. Histocompatibility typing may demonstrate HLA-DD, HLA-DR3, or HLA-DR4 antigens. Minor salivary gland biopsy is often performed for histopathologic confirmation of the clinical diagnosis.

  e. **Treatment:** Treatment of Sjögren's syndrome is symptomatic and supportive. Artificial tears and saliva may be of use in some patients, and steroids may help reduce the enlargement of the parotid glands. Radiation of the salivary glands has been implicated in the development of lymphoma and is therefore inappropriate in these patients. Active and consistent dental care and daily fluoride therapy are necessary to prevent caries.

C. **Inflammatory disorders**
  1. **Necrotizing sialometaplasia**
     a. **Chief complaint:** Painless ulceration on the palate.
     b. **Clinical features:** Necrotizing sialometaplasia is an inflammatory reaction of the salivary gland tissue. It may present as an area of ulceration, often bilateral, of the hard and soft palates, and can also occur on the buccal mucosa, lips, and retromolar region. These lesions typically are painless. Male patients are affected more often than female patients, and the lesions occur most often in the fourth and fifth decades of life. The ulceration and associated metaplasia are secondary to idiopathic ischemia, which clinically and histologically mimics malignancy.
     c. **Treatment:** The ulceration is self-limiting and heals by secondary intention.
  2. **Sialadenitis**
     See Chapter 7, "Facial Swellings."
D. **Salivary gland tumors**
  1. **Benign tumors**
     a. **Monomorphic adenoma**
        (1) **Chief complaint:** Painless mass in the upper lip.
        (2) **Clinical features:** Monomorphic adenoma

has a predilection for the major salivary glands and the upper lip. The lesion is characteristically found in older patients (median age 60 years), with a 5:1 predilection for occurrence in males, and is usually slow growing. The tumor has a clinical appearance consistent with a mucocele when it occurs in the upper lip.

(3) **Treatment:** Simple surgical excision is the treatment of choice for monomorphic adenoma, and recurrence is unlikely.

b. **Pleomorphic adenoma**

(1) **Chief complaint:** Small painless nodule in a major or minor salivary gland.

(2) **Clinical features:** Pleomorphic adenoma is the most common neoplasm of the major salivary glands. Approximately 85% to 90% of cases occur in the parotid gland, especially in the superficial lobe of the gland lateral to the facial nerve. The tumor can occur in any of the major or minor salivary glands. The lesion, which occurs with slightly greater frequency in female patients, is usually a painless, slow-growing nodule, with intermittent enlargement. The tumor is most common in the major salivary glands in the fourth to sixth decades of life and in the minor glands in the fifth to seventh decades. Major salivary gland pleomorphic adenomas are movable, nodular, round masses, usually without pain or paresis of the facial nerve.

Intraoral lesions account for a small percentage of these tumors, and tend to be less than 2 cm in diameter. The most common sites for intraoral pleomorphic adenomas are the palate and the lips. Since intraoral tumors tend to interfere with function, they usually are diagnosed and treated early, and thus are less likely to attain the size of the extraoral tumors.

Pleomorphic adenoma is capable of

malignant transformation, often in the untreated lesion of long duration or in instances of multiple recurrences.

(3) **Treatment:** Tumors in the parotid gland
are treated with lobectomy and preservation
of the facial nerve. In the submandibular
and sublingual glands the tumor is treated
by removal of the entire gland. Intraoral
tumors are treated by local surgical excision.

c. **Oncocytoma**

(1) **Chief complaint:** Lump in the parotid
gland, often of long duration.

(2) **Clinical features:** Oncocytoma is an uncommon benign tumor, small (typically 3 to
5 cm in diameter) and slow-growing. The
most common site of occurrence is the parotid gland. Patients are usually at least 50
years of age; women are more commonly
affected than men. The lesion is painless,
and its clinical features do not differentiate
this tumor from other benign salivary gland
tumors.

(3) **Treatment:** Surgical excision is the treatment of choice for oncocytoma, and recurrence is rare.

d. **Warthin's tumor (papillary cystadenoma
lymphomatosum)**

(1) **Chief complaint:** Mass in the parotid
gland.

(2) **Clinical features:** Warthin's tumor is found
predominantly in middle-aged men (5:1
compared with women). The tumor is well
encapsulated, usually superficial, painless,
and firm to doughy on palpation. It is invariably found in the parotid gland, and
may be bilateral in about 7% of patients.
These lesions are usually 3 to 4 cm in diameter by the time the clinical diagnosis is
made. Warthin's tumor is clinically indistinguishable from other benign tumors of
the salivary glands.

      (3) **Treatment:** Complete surgical excision is usually curative; recurrences are rare.

2. **Malignant tumors**

  a. **Acinic cell carcinoma**

    (1) **Chief complaint:** Mass in the parotid gland.

    (2) **Clinical features:** Acinic cell carcinoma is found primarily in the parotid gland, but may occur in the other major salivary glands or minor intraoral glands. The lesion tends to be slow-growing and painless, and may appear encapsulated. Typical intraoral sites include the lips and buccal mucosa. This tumor is predominantly found in middle age, and occasionally is bilateral.

    (3) **Treatment:** Wide surgical excision is recommended for this tumor, with variable recurrence rate. Because the tumor may recur many years after primary treatment, long-term follow-up care is indicated.

  b. **Adenoid cystic carcinoma**

    (1) **Chief complaint:** Mass in a major salivary gland, or small intraoral mass.

    (2) **Clinical features:** Adenoid cystic carcinoma is a malignant tumor of salivary gland origin, characterized by slow growth, pain, facial nerve (VII) paresis (when the parotid gland is involved by the tumor), local invasion, and fixation of the tumor mass. The most common sites of occurrence are the parotid and submaxillary glands, whereas in the mouth the tumor is most often discovered on the palate and in the tongue. Oral lesions are commonly ulcerated, and the tumor is notorious for early invasion of the perineural spaces. The tumor appears most frequently in the fifth and sixth decades of life. Clinically, the lesion may mimic a benign lesion of salivary gland tissue. The tumor metastasizes late in the course of the disease, with distant spread to the lungs, bone, and brain.

(3) **Treatment:** Wide surgical excision including resection of the underlying bone is the treatment of choice when the lesion occurs in the oral cavity. Radiation therapy in association with the surgical treatment plan may be appropriate. Close follow-up over prolonged periods is warranted. The lesion should not be considered controlled until the patient has been free of disease for at least a decade. The long-term prognosis for cure is guarded.

c. **Malignant pleomorphic adenoma**

(1) **Chief complaint:** Sudden growth in a long-standing mass of the parotid gland or on the palate.

(2) **Clinical features:** This tumor may represent malignant degeneration of a long-standing pleomorphic adenoma or de novo development of a primary malignant neoplasm. Patients with this tumor are usually a decade older than those with benign pleomorphic adenoma. The lesion may remain quiescent for a long time prior to a sudden increase in size associated with cervical lymphadenopathy. The primary sites of occurrence are the parotid glands, and intraorally on the palate. The tumor is often painful, larger than the typical benign form, fixed to the surrounding tissues, and may have surface ulceration.

(3) **Treatment:** The treatment of choice is wide surgical excision followed by radiation therapy. Local recurrence and distant metastasis to the lungs, bone, viscera, and brain are common.

d. **Mucoepidermoid carcinoma**

(1) **Chief complaint:** Mass in the parotid gland, or a palatal, lingual, or retromolar pad lesion.

(2) **Clinical features:** Mucoepidermoid carcinoma comprises less than 10% of all sali-

vary gland tumors but more than one third of all salivary gland malignancies. The primary area of occurrence is in the parotid gland. It occurs predominantly in the third to fifth decades of life, but has been reported in all age groups. There is a slight female predilection. The tumor has been divided into low-grade, intermediate, and high-grade histologic forms. The low-grade variety often simulates the pleomorphic adenoma; the high-grade form is characterized by rapid growth, facial nerve involvement, and pain. The tumors are usually less than 5 cm in diameter in the major salivary glands. The average duration reported before treatment is 1 to 1½ years.

Intraoral tumors are noted chiefly on the palate and retromolar area. The tumor is typically asymptomatic intraorally, and may feel cystlike because of the accumulation of mucoid material within the tumor. The lesion may be mistaken for a mucous retention phenomenon or other benign condition.

(3) **Treatment:** The definitive treatment of mucoepidermoid carcinoma is determined by its histologic type and clinical characteristics. Low-grade tumors are treated by wide surgical excision and long-term follow-up; more aggressive forms of the lesion require extensive surgical resection, and potentially regional lymph node dissection with postoperative radiation therapy. All patients with this tumor should be monitored closely for recurrences.

e. **Squamous cell carcinoma**
  (1) **Chief complaint:** Mass in a major salivary gland.
  (2) **Clinical features:** This uncommon malignancy of salivary gland tissue appears to be of ductal origin. The prognosis is poor. The lesion is found predominantly in the major

salivary glands, especially in patients who have received ionizing radiation to areas encompassing the affected glands. Local recurrences of squamous cell carcinoma with regional lymph node metastasis are to be anticipated, and may be part of the presenting symptom complex. Specific clinical findings limited to this clinicopathologic entity are simply not available for description.

(3) **Treatment:** Wide surgical excision with radical neck dissection and adjuvant radiation therapy is indicated for this tumor. Local and distant recurrences of the tumor are common.

BIBLIOGRAPHY

Batsakis JG: *Tumors of the Head and Neck,* ed 2. Baltimore, Williams & Wilkins, 1979.

Cawson RA, Eveson JW: *Oral Pathology and Diagnosis.* Philadelphia, WB Saunders, 1987.

Donoff BR: *Manual of Oral and Maxillofacial Surgery.* St Louis, CV Mosby, 1987.

Eversole LR: *Clinical Outline of Oral Pathology: Diagnosis and Treatment,* ed 2. Philadelphia, Lea & Febiger, 1984.

Peterson LJ, Ellis E, Hupp JR, et al: *Contemporary Oral and Maxillofacial Surgery.* St Louis, CV Mosby, 1988.

Rankow RM, Polayes IM: *Diseases of the Salivary Glands.* Philadelphia, WB Saunders, 1976.

Regezi JA, Sciubba JJ: *Oral Pathology: Clinical-Pathologic Correlations.* Philadelphia, WB Saunders, 1989.

Shafer WG, Hine MK, Levy BM: *Textbook of Oral Pathology,* ed 4. Philadelphia, WB Saunders, 1983.

Wood NK, Goaz PA: *Differential Diagnosis of Oral Lesions,* ed 4. St Louis, CV Mosby, 1975.

Chapter 6 _____

Temporomandibular Disorders

Daniel M. Laskin
Raymond F. Zambito

_____

The term **temporomandibular joint (TMJ) disorder** often is used erroneously to describe a condition in which the joint itself is not the primary source of the dysfunction. Musculoskeletal disorders, rather than joint disease, frequently prove to be the source of symptoms and complaints in the jaw or in referred areas of the head and neck. These complaints may include pain in the face, neck, shoulders, and back; headache; inability to find a restful jaw position; difficulty in opening the mouth; and pain on chewing.

Temporomandibular disorder (TMD) is the preferred umbrella term, with subdivision into true joint disease (TMJ) and myofascial pain/dysfunction (MPD) syndrome.

The first step in diagnosis therefore involves determining whether the problem is **intracapsular** (TMJ) or **extracapsular** (muscular). This distinction is not always easy, because both intracapsular and extracapsular conditions may cause the same

129

dysfunctional complaints. Much of the confusion existent in the management of TMD relates to the failure to make this distinction and, as a result, treating what is really a variety of etiologically unrelated conditions in a similar manner.

I. HISTORY OF TEMPOROMANDIBULAR DISORDERS

As early as 1918, Prentiss theorized that vertical collapse of the occlusion was responsible for TMJ pain/dysfunction. Later this was supported by Costen (Costen's syndrome). A concentration on occlusion persisted into the late 1950s, when Schwartz, based on his experiences at Columbia University, suggested that the problem involved the masticatory muscles rather than the joint, that there was a multifactorial dimension to the myofascial pain and dysfunction, and that occlusion played a minor role as the primary cause, although it might be a contributing factor. Until that time the approach to management of TMD generally was a one-disease one-treatment concept, and that treatment usually involved alterations in the occlusion. Schwartz's approach brought to the fore the idea that all patients were not to be treated the same.

In 1969 attention was focused on the muscular component of TMD, when the psychophysiologic theory of **myofascial pain/dysfunction (MPD) syndrome** was described. Since then extensive research has been conducted to establish and identify more critically the multifactorial causes contributing to TMD. This had led to a better understanding of the problem and improved care of patients. The reader is directed to the many library sources and to the literature regarding such information.

II. DIAGNOSIS

A. Major categories of temporomandibular disorders

Although the TMJ is heir to the same problems as other joints of the body, the solutions are often different. Most other joint problems are solved surgically; most temporomandibular pain and dysfunction problems are solved nonsurgically. The TMJ is distinct from other joints because (1) both joints function as one unit; (2) the joint contains an important growth site for the mandible, which is basically unprotected; other bones have their growth sites farther down in the epiphyseal region; and (3) the relationship of the articulating components is influenced by the dentition. Temporomandibular disorders fall into one of two major categories: either a form of true joint disease or a masticatory muscle problem. In addition there is a large group of extra-articular problems that may mimic these conditions, and which must be taken into consideration in the differential diagnosis. Thus pain or limitation of mandibular motion may fit into one of three diagnostic groups:

1. a. **Extra-articular causes of jaw pain**
   (1) Pulpitis
   (2) Pericoronitis
   (3) Otitis
   (4) Parotitis
   (5) Sinusitis
   (6) Trigeminal neuralgia
   (7) Atypical (vascular) neuralgia
   (8) Temporal arteritis
   (9) Trotter's syndrome (nasopharyngeal carcinoma)
   (10) Eagle syndrome (elongated styloid process)

   b. **Extra-articular causes of jaw limitation/dysfunction**
   (1) Odontogenic infection
   (2) Nonodontogenic infection
   (3) Myositis
   (4) Myositis ossificans
   (5) Neoplasia
   (6) Scleroderma
   (7) Hysteria
   (8) Tetanus
   (9) Extrapyramidal reactions
   (10) Depressed zygomatic arch
   (11) Osteochondroma of coronoid process

2. **Myofascial pain/dysfunction (MPD) syndrome**
3. **True intracapsular disease**

When those patients with extra-articular causes of jaw pain and dysfunction are excluded, about 15% to 20% of the remaining patients fall into the group with true TMJ disease, and the remaining 80% to 85% have MPD syndrome.

B. Differential diagnosis of TMJ disease
  1. Congenital and developmental anomalies:
    a. Agenesis.
    b. Hypoplasia.
    c. Hyperplasia.
  2. Traumatic injuries:
    a. Dislocation.
    b. Fracture.
  3. Ankylosis.
  4. Neoplasia.
  5. Arthritis:
    a. Infectious.
    b. Traumatic.
    c. Rheumatoid.
    d. Degenerative.
  6. Internal derangement.
C. Diagnostic workup
  The following information is important in establishing a correct diagnosis:
  1. History of present illness:
    a. **Time of onset of pain,** and what may have caused it.
    b. **Duration of pain.** Determination of whether the pain is acute or chronic. (Pain persisting 6 months or longer is considered chronic pain.)
    c. **Exact location of pain.** The patient is asked to use one finger to point to the painful area. Usually in MPD syndrome the patient is unable to use one finger to point to the painful area and will use the hand to identify a radiant distribution pattern. With joint disease the patient can usually indicate the precise region.
    d. **Description of the pain.** A sharp, lancinating pain generally indicates nerve involvement. Aching or gnawing pain generally arises from mus-

cle, bone, or tendon. Burning, throbbing pain usually has a vascular origin. Pulpal pain generally is diffuse, whereas periodontal pain usually is very discretely identified, because the periodontal structures have proprioceptive receptors, whereas pulpal tissue does not.

e. **When is the pain better?** Request a complete description of what the patient does to diminish the pain.

f. **When is the pain worse?** For example, does time of day, body position, or activity cause a change?

g. **Onset of jaw limitation/dysfunction** and its subsequent course.

h. **What previous therapy,** if any, has been administered? What has been the response?

i. **Has the patient seen other clinicians?** If so, what was the diagnosis?

2. **Clinical examination:**

a. **Check for range of mandibular movement.** Measure interincisal opening and degree of protrusive and lateral movement in millimeters.

b. **Examine the TMJs** during these movements.

c. **Palpate the joint and auscultate** it for noise through a stethoscope.

d. **Examine the ear and eardrum.**

e. **Palpate the masticatory muscles bimanually,** especially the masseter and temporalis and the cervical and shoulder muscles.

f. **Examine the dentition** for evidence of parafunctional habits, such as clenching and grinding.

g. **Examine the occlusion.**

h. **Perform the tongue blade test.** Have the patient bite on a tongue blade placed between the posterior teeth on one side, then on the contralateral side. Ask the patient to explain how this affects the pain. If the pain is of joint origin, biting on the side opposite the pain causes loading of the involved joint and the pain is worse; if the pain is of muscular origin, biting on the same side as the pain will make the pain worse.

3. **Imaging techniques:**
   a. **Screening films,** such as panoramic or transcranial radiographs, should be used when bony joint disease is suspected. These radiographs are used only to detect gross bone disease. Condylar position and characteristics of the joint space cannot be accurately ascertained using transcranial radiographs.
   b. **Corrected polycycloidal tomography or computed tomography** should be used if screening films demonstrate bony changes.
   c. **Magnetic resonance imaging** (MRI) or arthrography coupled with cinefluorography should be used to visualize the intra-articular disc.
4. **Laboratory tests** (limited value):
   a. **Complete blood cell count** and differential cell count can be used if an infection is suspected.
   b. **Erythrocyte sedimentation rate** can be used to monitor the course of rheumatoid arthritis but not as a diagnostic test.
   c. **Tests for rheumatoid arthritis** include rheumatoid factor, latex fixation, and antinuclear antibody tests.
5. **Other studies:**
   a. **Radionuclide uptake studies** (technetium, gallium).
   b. **Diagnostic arthroscopy.**

III. **ETIOLOGY AND THERAPY**
   A. **Intrinsic joint disease**
      The three most common types of intrinsic joint disease that produce pain and limitation of jaw movement are rheumatoid arthritis, degenerative joint disease, and internal disc derangement.
      1. **Rheumatoid arthritis**
         The medical literature reports that 50% of patients with rheumatoid arthritis have TMJ involvement. Rheumatoid arthritis can be clinically silent even though there is disease within the joint.
         a. **Signs and symptoms** of rheumatoid arthritis include:
            (1) Intermittent joint pain and swelling.
            (2) Limitation of motion, often progressive.

(3) Usually, involvement of both TMJs.

(4) Generally, involvement of other joints (e.g., wrists, hands, ankles, spine).

(5) Presence of anemia, fever, malaise, and anorexia.

(6) Positive laboratory test results (rheumatoid factor, latex fixation, antinuclear antibody).

(7) Late radiographic changes, including erosion of the condyle and osteophyte formation.

Rheumatoid arthritis is not a primary disease of bone but is a disease of synovial tissues. Therefore, when condylar changes are seen on radiographs it is usually late in the course of the disease.

When there is extensive destruction of the condyle an open bite may be one of the patient's complaints. In children, rheumatoid arthritis may have secondary effects on mandibular growth and midface structure.

Often observation of the patient's fingers and wrists can help establish a diagnosis of rheumatoid arthritis. With rheumatoid arthritis the midphalangeal joint is widened, causing the fingers to be spindle shaped; there is ulnar deviation of the hand and fingers; and the patient has a weak grip.

b. Therapy for rheumatoid arthritis includes:

(1) **Primary medical management.**

(2) **Preventive dental care** is strongly urged, because limitation of jaw motion can progress and make dental treatment difficult.

(3) **Surgical correction of ankylosis** may be indicated when mandibular movement is greatly restricted.

(4) **Orthognathic surgery** may be required when there is facial deformity or open bite.

2. **Degenerative joint disease**

In degenerative joint disease the terminal interphalangeal joints are involved, and the fingers are knobby but straight.

a. Types:

(1) **Primary:**

a. Relatively asymptomatic; some crepitation may be present.

    b. Occurs in elderly patients (60 to 80 years of age) and is part of the aging process.

  (2) Secondary:
    a. Symptomatic.
    b. Occurs in younger patients.
    c. Caused by macrotrauma or can result from chronic bruxing and clenching, as occurs in some patients with MPD syndrome.

b. Signs and symptoms:
 (1) Constant dull, aching pain in preauricular region.
 (2) Pain is well localized.
 (3) TMJ is tender to both lateral and intrameatal palpation.
 (4) Occasional masticatory muscular tenderness due to reflex splinting of the jaw.
 (5) Mild to moderate limitation of motion.
 (6) Crepitant sounds in the later stages.

c. Radiographic changes are possible in the later stages, and include:
 (1) Subchondral sclerosis.
 (2) Marginal lipping.
 (3) Condylar flattening (condyle looks like a mushroom rather than a bean).
 (4) Surface erosion and osteophyte formation.
 (5) Bone cysts (Ely's cyst).
 (6) Decreased joint space, indicative of disc damage.
 (7) Changes in the articular eminence.

d. Treatment:
 (1) Nonsteroidal anti-inflammatory drugs (NSAIDs) or aspirin in high doses. It is important to titrate the dosage, because all of these drugs are flat plane, or ceiling, drugs.
 (2) Muscle relaxing drugs if muscle spasm is present.
 (3) Rest of the mandible.
 (4) Moist heat.

  (5) Soft diet.

  (6) Excellent dental care to eliminate any contributing factors.

  (7) Surgery as a last resort.

    Degenerative joint disease usually is arrested, not cured. The patient is taught how to manage the disease medically.

3. Internal derangement of TMJ:

An internal derangement is an abnormal relationship between the disc and the condyle when the teeth are in occlusion. Figure 6–1 shows the possible causes of internal derangements.

a. Types

 Internal derangements are classified as:

  (1) Incoordination (slight binding or catching sensation).

  (2) Anterior disc displacement with reduction (clicking).

  (3) Anterior disc displacement without reduction (locking).

  NOTE: The chronic clenching associated with MPD syndrome, over time, causes compression of the disc and articular structures,

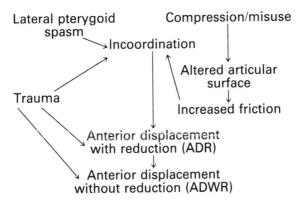

FIG 6–1.
Causes of internal derangement of TMJ.

changes in the lubrication and frictional properties of the joint, and ultimately alteration in the articular surfaces and disc displacement.

b. **Treatment**

Nonsurgical treatment of the clicking joint involves:

(a) Relief of pain with NSAIDs.

(b) Control of parafunctional habits.

(c) Use of bite opening or anterior repositioning appliances.

The intent of the bite opening appliance is to keep the teeth from occluding and thereby keep the disc "recaptured." Anterior repositioning appliances assist in recapturing the disc by bringing the mandible forward. These appliances are worn 24 hours a day for 1 to 2 months, with the intent of allowing healing to keep the disc permanently in place. Appliance therapy helps only about 15% to 20% of patients, because in most instances the condition is chronic and repair is not possible.

If the patient has only residual clicking, observation is recommended. However, if the patient has continued pain and clicking despite nonsurgical therapy, surgery is generally indicated. Surgery is also indicated for patients with anterior disc displacement without reduction. Surgical treatment for clicking involves discoplasty done either arthroscopically or via arthrotomy. When the disc does not recapture on opening (locking), an attempt at discoplasty should still be made. If the disc is not salvageable, discectomy with alloplastic or autogenous replacement should be done.

B. Myofascial Pain/Dysfunction Syndrome

Myofascial pain/dysfunction (MPD) syndrome is a psychophysiologic disease. The source of the problem lies in the muscles of mastication, which are in spasm. The most common cause of the myospasm is muscular fatigue resulting from hyperactivity either centrally generated or related to chronic bruxism. Other causes of myospasm are muscular overextension (excessive opening of the bite) and muscular overcontraction (overclosure of the bite) (Fig 6–2).

In the early stages MPD syndrome is a functional disorder. However, if the condition persists long enough, muscle disease, joint disease, and in some patients occlusal dysharmony can develop. MPD syndrome affects women more frequently than men; the ratio varies from 3:1 to 5:1. The greatest incidence is in the 20 to 40 years age group.

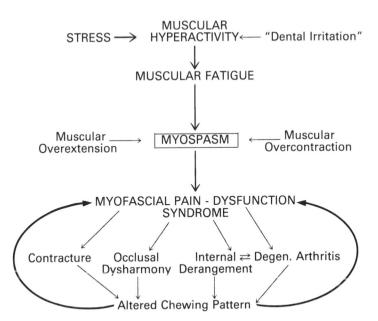

FIG 6–2.
Etiology of myofascial pain/dysfunction syndrome. (Modified from Laskin DM: *J Am Dent Assoc* 1969; 79:147.)

The signs and symptoms of MPD syndrome include:

1. **Dull, aching, radiating pain** that is not well localized.
2. **No joint tenderness** on lateral or intrameatal palpation.
3. **Moderate to severe limitation of motion.**
4. **Muscle tenderness,** which is usually unilateral and involves the masticatory and cervical muscles. The masseter muscle is most commonly involved, followed by the temporalis, medial pterygoid, and lateral pterygoid muscles. Tenderness in these muscles is often at the site of tendinous attachment.
5. **Clicking and popping sounds.**
6. **No radiographic changes** in the TMJ.
1. **Therapy of MPD syndrome**
   a. **General**
      The following rules should be observed in the treatment of MPD syndrome:
      (1) **Avoid irreversible therapy,** including surgery, injection of local anesthetics and steroids into muscles, multiple steroid injections into the joint, and inappropriate equilibration of teeth or placement of onlays or crowns.
      (2) **Use escalation therapy.** Start with the simplest form of treatment, and escalate only if necessary.
      (3) **Consider the placebo effect** and the effect of the doctor-patient relationship on the efficacy of therapy.
      (4) **Emphasize management rather than cure,** because, in a sense, a psychophysiologic disease is not curable.
      (5) **Use a team approach** for treatment of the difficult patient. Include those members of the healing professions who supplement your area of expertise.
   b. **Specific**
      There are four phases of treatment in keeping with the concept of escalation of therapy.

Phase 1.—Phase 1 generally lasts 2 to 4 weeks
  a. Give the patient an **initial explanation of the problem and its physiologic basis.** It is generally not advisable to discuss psychologic factors at this point.
  b. **Prescribe home therapy.** This includes a conscious effort by the patient to avoid clenching; the adverse effects of parafunctional habits must be stressed. A soft, nonchewy diet; limitation of jaw motion; and the use of moist heat and muscle massage are recommended.
  c. **Prescribe muscle relaxant and analgesic drugs.** Generally, this involves small doses (2 to 5 mg) of diazepam and a nonsteroidal anti-inflammatory drug such as ibuprofen (400 to 600 mg 3 to 4 times daily).
About 50% of patients will be helped by phase 1 therapy.

Phase 2.—Phase 2 usually lasts another 2 to 4 weeks. If no improvement was noted in phase 1:
  a. **Reevaluate the diagnosis.**
  b. **Check patient compliance** in the proper use of diet, limitation of movement, heat and massage, and medications. If lack of compliance is suspected, suggest that the patient keep a diary.
  c. **Continue home therapy and medications.**
  d. **Fabricate a bite appliance.** This represents an escalation of therapy. The recommended appliance for MPD syndrome is a maxillary acrylic appliance (Hawley or Sved type) with a flat, nonguiding anterior platform that creates minimal opening (1 to 2 mm) of the bite. The appliance is worn at night, and can also be used for 3 to 4 hours a day if necessary. If the appliance is effective, discontinue the use of medications.

Approximately 70% of the patients will be helped by phases 1 and 2 of therapy.

Phase 3.—For the 30% of patients who are not helped by phases 1 and 2 of therapy, further escalation of treatment for 4 to 6 weeks is recommended, as follows:

   a. **Continue home therapy and medications.**
   b. **Reevaluate the bite appliance.**
   c. **Initiate physical therapy** (ultrasound, electrogalvanic stimulation, and mild active stretching exercises).
   d. **Use relaxation treatment** (either biofeedback or conditioned relaxation).

It is recommended that physical therapy and relaxation therapy not be introduced at the same time, but consecutively, if necessary. There is no evidence that one treatment is more efficacious than the other, although the patient may have a personal preference. Phase 3 therapy should help another 20% of patients; for the remaining 10%, escalate to phase 4.

Phase 4.—Phase 4 therapy includes the following:

   a. **Reevaluate the diagnosis and patient compliance** thoroughly.
   b. **Seek consultation** from medical colleagues (ENT, Neurology) if this has not been done previously.
   c. **Recommend psychologic counseling.**
   d. **Refer the patient to a pain center.**

2. **Termination of therapy**

When it is determined that MPD syndrome is under control, termination of therapy is in order. When treatment in any phase has been successful: (1) phase out treatment; (2) give the patient a final, detailed explanation of the problem; (3) give instructions for self-management; and (4) offer the patient a follow-up appointment.

The final explanation of the problem to the patient should emphasize:

1. MPD syndrome is a psychophysiologic disorder, similar to an ulcer.
2. The symptoms are not imaginary.
3. Stress may cause the symptoms.
4. Stressors in the patient's life need to be identified.
5. The patient needs to learn how to manage the condition.

IV. SUMMARY

The successful management of temporomandibular disorders depends on establishing an accurate diagnosis and understanding the cause of the problem. Establishing an accurate diagnosis is accomplished through a careful history, thorough clinical examination, and knowledge of the signs and symptoms of the various conditions.

It is important to remember that MPD syndrome is a psychophysiologic disease and that therapy should be directed at reducing stress, relaxing tense jaw muscles, and making patients conscious of the cause of the problem and their role in correcting or controlling it. Only reversible forms of therapy are recommended.

In the management of all temporomandibular disorders, thorough evaluation of the problem, careful execution of therapy, and understanding the role of the placebo effect and the doctor-patient relationship lead to most effective therapy.

BIBLIOGRAPHY

Ireland VE: The problem of "the clicking jaw." Proc R Soc Med 1951; 44:363–372.

Laskin DM: Etiology of the pain-dysfunction syndrome. *J Am Dent Assoc* 1969; 79:147.

Laskin DM, Block S: Diagnosis and treatment of myofascial pain-dysfunction (MPD) syndrome. *J Prosthet Dent* 1986; 56:75–84.

McNeill C (ed): *Craniomandibular Disorders: Guidelines for Evaluation, Diagnosis, and Management*. Chicago, Quintessence, 1990.

Travell JG, Simons DG: *Myofascial Pain and Dysfunction: The Trigger Point Manual*. Baltimore, Williams & Wilkins, 1983.

Facial Swellings

Anthony J. Casino

     A. Sialadenitis/Sialolithiasis
     B. Ranula
     C. Dacryorhinocystitis
VI. Congenital/Developmental Swelling
     A. Cystic Hygroma
     B. Masseteric Hypertrophy
     C. Facial Asymmetry
     D. Fibrous Dysplasia
VII. Traumatic/Postsurgical Swelling
     A. Edema
     B. Hematoma
     C. Infection

Swelling of the face and contiguous anatomic structures (e.g., neck) is manifested by alteration in normal anatomic form; facial symmetry is used as a guide in determining the change in form. Occasionally facial swelling occurs bilaterally. Swelling may cause dysfunction of anatomic systems.

The causes of facial swelling are varied, and can be classified as:

1. Inflammatory
2. Infectious
3. Neoplastic
4. Cystic
5. Obstructive/retentive
6. Congenital/developmental
7. Traumatic/surgical

The mechanism by which a change of normal anatomy occurs can be attributed to an increase in tissue mass (neoplastic, congenital, cystic) or to an increase in the products of cellular function (inflammatory, obstructive/retentive, infectious).

Determining the cause of facial swelling utilizes the principles of **physical diagnosis** (see Chapter 1). A good rule in the process of diagnosis is to begin with the anatomic location of the swelling. This distinction will allow an excellent guide to the cause of the lesion. For example, swellings of the preauricular region usually represent disease of the **parotid gland.**

After determination of the anatomic region of the lesion, the next phase is to classify the swelling. The major categorization will be made between **inflammatory/infectious** lesions and **cystic/neoplastic/congenital** lesions. This process is easily aided by factoring in the **symptoms, physical examination,** and **history.** At this point, **radiography, laboratory tests,** and **tissue diagnostic techniques** are considered means to definitive diagnosis.

I. INFLAMMATORY SWELLING
Characteristics of inflammatory swelling include:
1. Rapid onset
2. Erythema
3. Pain
4. Systemic symptoms
5. Fever
6. Local temperature change
7. Precipitating factors (allergy)
8. Drainage

Inflammatory swellings of the face include:
1. Angioneurotic edema
2. Sjögren's syndrome
3. Sarcoidosis (parotid)
4. Obstructive sialadenitis
5. Cheilitis granulomatosa
6. Erythema multiforme
7. Allergic reactions
8. Cat-scratch disease

A. Angioneurotic edema
1. **History:** Rapid onset of diffuse facial swelling. May be due to allergy to certain foods or drugs or to endocrine disturbance. Hereditary form of angioneurotic edema caused by deficiency of C1 esterase inhibitor.
2. **Anatomic location:** Face, primarily around the lips, chin, eyes, and tongue.
3. **Symptoms:** Tense, diffuse swelling of the facial region. Usually not painful. May cause acute anxiety, especially when combined with possible airway involvement.
4. **Physical examination:** Although diffuse, swelling in angioneurotic edema is soft and the skin usually is not erythematous.

5. **Treatment:** Avoid or withdraw suspected etiologic agent or substance.
   a. **Antihistamine:** Diphenhydramine (Benadryl) 50 mg PO IV stat, then 25 mg PO q6h until swelling subsides.
   b. **Hereditary form** should be determined by medical workup. **Fresh frozen plasma** has been used as prophylaxis prior to exposure to suspected allergens (e.g., local anesthetics, or stressful surgery or trauma).

B. **Sjögren's syndrome**
   1. **History:** Unilateral or bilateral swelling of the parotid or submandibular glands. Xerostomia, xerophthalmia, and rheumatoid arthritis or another connective tissue disease constitute Sjögren's syndrome.
   2. **Anatomic location:** Preauricular and/or submandibular gland enlargement.
   3. **Symptoms:** Swelling, along with xerostomia and conjunctivitis sicca. Pain may be present.
   4. **Physical examination:** Nontender enlargement of the salivary glands, with reduced salivary flow.
   5. **Radiographic/laboratory tests:**
      a. LE prep.
      b. Rheumatoid factor.
      c. Antinuclear antibodies.
      d. Salivary flow rate.
      e. Sialography.
   6. **Tissue diagnostic techniques:** Minor salivary gland biopsy of the palatal or labial minor mucous glands to examine histologically for periductal lymphocytic infiltrates.
   7. **Treatment:**
      a. **Symptomatic:**
         (1) Artificial saliva.
         (2) Artificial tears.
         (3) Topical fluoride treatment.
         (4) Dental care and routine recall.
      b. Radiation and/or surgery only in extreme cases.
      c. Workup and follow-up for **lymphoma.**

C. **Sarcoidosis (parotid)**
   1. **History:** Benign disease of unknown cause; usually self-limiting, with insidious onset and protracted course.
   2. **Anatomic location:** Pulmonary lesions are the most common sites of granuloma formation. Other involved areas include skin, eyes, liver, bone, and parotid gland.
   3. **Symptoms:** Fever, gastrointestinal disturbances, arthralgia, and night sweats sometime precede parotid gland involvement. Swelling may be unilateral or bilateral.
   4. **Diagnosis:** A differential diagnosis must be made to rule out other forms of parotid gland enlargement. Specific techniques of distinguishing sarcoid include (1) presence of other organ involvement and (2) **Kveim test.** Biopsy of the mass provides the final diagnosis.
   5. **Treatment:** Mainly supportive. Corticosteroids are the drugs of choice during the active stages. Secondary xerostomia may require treatment with artificial saliva, and fluoride treatment to prevent dental caries.
D. **Obstructive sialadenitis**
   See "Sialadenitis," section II E.
E. **Cheilitis granulomatosa**
   1. **History:** Gradual diffuse swelling of the lips.
   2. **Anatomic location:** Lips, particularly the lower lip.
   3. **Symptoms:** Pain is usually absent. Swelling is diffuse, but sometimes nodular.
   4. **Physical examination:** Diffuse, sometimes nodular, swelling of the lips, without erythema of the surface tissues.
   5. **Tissue diagnostic techniques:** Incisional biopsy is sometimes performed.
   6. **Treatment:** Injection with **steroids** causes reduction of swelling.
F. **Erythema multiforme** (including Stevens-Johnson syndrome)
   1. **History:** Acute eruptions of the oral cavity and lips, causing vesicles and ulcerations. Pain and

swelling are the rule. Stevens-Johnson syndrome can be fatal.

2. **Anatomic location:** Skin, oral cavity, lips, eyes, and genitalia.

3. **Physical examination:** Oral mucous membrane eruptions of vesicles and ulcerations. May cause edema and lip enlargement. Eye lesions are also common, and include photophobia and conjunctivitis.

4. **Treatment:** Systemic signs of fever, dehydration, and malaise should be treated aggressively with IV fluids and steroids.

G. **Allergic reactions**

1. **History:** Patients may report acute facial edema following exposure to allergens similar to that in angioneurotic edema.

2. **Anatomic location:** Face, lips, and eyes.

3. **Physical examination:** Soft edematous swelling; may be erythematous.

4. **Treatment:** Reactions are usually type I immediate hypersensitivity reactions due to histamine release. Treatment consists of a course of antihistamines, such as **Diphenhydramine** (Benadryl) 25 mg PO qid. If the reaction is severe and compromises the airway, then **Epinephrine** 0.3 to 0.5 mg IM/IV/SC.

H. **Cat-scratch disease**

1. **History:** Swelling of cervical lymph nodes of the neck and occasionally submandibular region 1 to 3 weeks after a scratch or bite by a household cat.

2. **Anatomic location:** Cervical and submandibular lymph nodes commonly affected.

3. **Symptoms:** Painful lymphadenopathy of affected areas. Fever may be present, accompanied by chills, nausea, malaise, and headache.

4. **Physical examination:** Tender lymph nodes, with overlying erythema of the skin. Lymph nodes may be large, freely moveable, and warm.

5. **Treatment:** Symptomatic management; incision and drainage of sterile lymph node abscesses may be necessary.

II. INFECTIOUS SWELLING (bacterial, viral, fungal)

Characteristics of infectious swelling include:

1. Rapid onset
2. Erythema
3. Pain
4. Systemic symptoms
5. Fever
6. Local temperature change
7. Precipitating factors (allergy)
8. Drainage

Infectious swellings of the face include:

1. Cellulitis
2. Abscess (space infection)
3. Actinomycosis
4. Lymphadenitis
5. Sialadenitis
6. Endemic parotitis (mumps)
7. Tuberculosis (scrofula)
8. Acute sinusitis
9. Infectious mononucleosis

NOTE: For a discussion of infections of dental etiology, see Chapter 2, "Odontogenic Infections."

A. Cellulitis

1. **History:** Cellulitis is gradual or rapid swelling of the face or jaws caused by an infectious process. Cellulitis is diffuse and nonlocalized, and usually associated with pain. Cellulitis of the face and neck often results as a sequela of odontogenic infection, and spreads along fascial planes.

2. **Anatomic location:** Initially the cellulitis is contained within the area of the offending tooth, but can spread quickly via perforation of the cortical plates to involve anatomic spaces (canine, infratemporal, pterygomandibular, lateral pharyngeal, retropharyngeal, parotid, buccal, submandibular, submental, sublingual spaces). See Chapter 2 for additional descriptions of facial space infections.

   A specific type of cellulitis, **Ludwig's angina,** is the involvement of bilateral submandibular, sublingual, and submental spaces.

3. **Symptoms:** Swelling, pain, fever, trismus, and

dysphagia may be associated with dental or jaw pain and odontogenic infection.

4. **Physical examination:** The swelling in cellulitis is diffuse, causing the skin to be brawny and erythematous. The process sometimes becomes "pointed," with an area to be drained.

5. **Tissue diagnostic techniques:**
   a. Aspiration of infectious material (if present).
   b. Gram stain.
   c. Culture and sensitivity testing (aerobic and anaerobic).

6. **Treatment:**
   a. Accurate diagnosis.
   b. Appropriate antibiotics (if necessary).
   c. Drainage of abscess formation.
   d. Removal of cause.

B. **Abscess (space infection)**
   Swelling caused by infectious processes may become localized and wall itself off from the body by formation of an abscess. Occasionally abscesses are involved with deep spaces. The abscess cavity is difficult to detect. Superficial abscess presents as "fluctuant" swelling of intraoral and extraoral regions. Treatment includes drainage, antibiotic therapy, and removal of the etiologic agent.

C. **Actinomycosis**
   1. **History:** Gradual swelling of the lower face and/or neck. May be associated with fever and malaise.
   2. **Anatomic location:** Submandibular and lateral neck regions.
   3. **Symptoms:** Pain, gradual enlargement of affected region. Drainage may be via sinus tracts exiting on the skin surface.
   4. **Physical examination:** Indurated, nodular, and sometimes fluctuant swelling. Overlying skin may be red to purplish. Sinus tracts drain the classic **sulfur granules.**
   5. **Treatment:** Diagnosis is made by clinical signs and **culture.** Organism may be anaerobic and often difficult to culture. Use anaerobic culture medium when actinomycosis is suspected.

       a. Antibiotics: Long-term penicillin or tetracycline therapy is successful against actinomycosis.

       b. Rule out pulmonary and abdominal forms.

D. Lymphadenitis

   1. History: Acute enlargement of a "node" in the face or neck region.

   2. Anatomic location: Depends on the origin of the primary infection.

   3. Symptoms: Pain, swelling, dysphagia; fever may be present.

   4. Physical examination: Tender, painful swelling. Usually nodular enlargement. Lesions are firm, round, discrete, and moveable. Overlying erythema may be present, as well as multifocal node involvement.

   5. Treatment:

       a. Diagnose primary cause.

       b. Treat primary source of the infection.

       c. Antibiotics PO/IV, if indicated.

E. Sialadenitis

   1. History: Sialadenitis of the major salivary glands is characterized by painful swelling of the affected gland. Infection and swelling caused by obstruction may cause intermittent swelling at mealtime. Patients with decreased salivary flow have an increased tendency for sialadenitis. Sialadenitis may also be noted in patients with psychiatric disorders, alcoholism, or xerostomia and in patients with functioning xerostomia secondary to a wide variety of medications, including but not limited to diuretics, tranquilizers, antidepressants, and antihypertensives.

   2. Anatomic location: Submandibular triangle when infections involve the submandibular gland; preauricular region when swelling involves the parotid gland.

   3. Symptoms: Swelling of submandibular triangle or preauricular region. May be exacerbated by meals. Erythema may be present over the gland if swelling is severe. Area is usually tender to palpation.

4. **Radiographic/laboratory findings:**
   a. Leukocytosis.
   b. Increased serum amylase level (salivary type).
   c. Salivary stones (sialoliths).
5. **Physical examination:** Swelling of the submandibular or preauricular region. May be associated with skin erythema and tenderness. There may be purulent discharge from Stensen's or Wharton's duct.
6. **Treatment:**
   a. Clinical examination and diagnosis.
   b. Occlusal and/or posteroanterior radiographs to rule out sialoliths (stones) of the submandibular or parotid duct.
   c. Culture and sensitivity testing of any purulent discharge.
   d. Hydration (may require hospital admission and IV fluids).
   e. Palpation and massage of ductal systems.
   f. If stones are absent, dilation of the ducts may be indicated to relieve blockage or to dilate a stricture to facilitate flow or drainage. Dilation is performed using lacrimal probe sizes 0000 to 2.
   g. **Broad-spectrum antibiotics:**
      (1) Dicloxicillin 500 mg PO qid for 7 days.
      (2) Cephalexin (Keflex) 500 mg PO qid for 7 days.

F. **Endemic parotitis (mumps)**
   1. **History:** Swelling of parotid glands; may be unilateral or bilateral. Preceded by headache, fever, chills, and vomiting. Usually occurs in children.
   2. **Anatomic location:** Parotid glands; 70% bilateral presentation.
   3. **Symptoms:** Parotid gland enlargement with pain, occurring at mealtime. Fever, chills, malaise.
   4. **Physical examination:** Bilateral or unilateral parotid swelling. Orifice of Stensen's duct may be inflamed.
   5. **Treatment:** Symptomatic. **Mumps vaccine** is available for use in children.

G. Tuberculosis (scrofula)
   1. **History:** Swelling of the submandibular and/or cervical lymph nodes. May be concomitant with active pulmonary tuberculosis.
   2. **Anatomic location:** Submandibular and/or cervical lymph nodes.
   3. **Symptoms:** Fever, malaise, chills, weight loss, painful swelling of the cervical lymph nodes.
   4. **Physical examination:** Lymph node swelling; nodes may be firm or fluctuant. Usually manifested by overlying erythema. Drainage and abscess formation may be present.
   5. **Diagnosis:**
      a. Diagnosis based on presence of lung lesions.
      b. Culture and sensitivity testing of drainage and/or sputum.
   6. **Treatment:**
      a. Antibiotic therapy.
H. Acute sinusitis
   1. **History:** May be preceded by a common upper respiratory tract infection or maxillary dental infection.
   2. **Anatomic location:** Unilateral or bilateral midfacial swelling in the infraorbital regions; may include lower eye lid and lateral nasal area.
   3. **Symptoms:** Pain, pressure, swelling of face and head. There may be associated congestion, nasal stuffiness, and postnasal drip or discharge.
   4. **Physical examination:** Swelling, tenderness to palpation of the anterior maxilla and malar regions. Tenderness to percussion of the maxillary teeth and lateral sinus wall. Discharge may be seen on nasal speculum examination.
   5. **Radiography:**
      a. Sinus series, posteroanterior and lateral.
      b. Water's view.
      c. Panoramic views.
      d. CT scan.
   6. **Diagnosis:** Clinical findings together with a cloudy or congested sinus on radiographic examination provide the information for accurate diagnosis.

7. **Treatment:**
   a. Culture and sensitivity testing of any purulent discharge.
   b. Broad-spectrum antibiotics effective against *Staphylococcus* and *Haemophilus influenzae:*
      (1) Ampicillin 500 mg PO qid.
      (2) Cephalosporin (Keflex) 500 mg PO qid.
   c. Decongestants:
      (1) Dimetapp Extentabs, 1 tablet PO tid.
      (2) Drixoral, 1 tablet PO tid.
   d. Nasal decongestant spray (Afrin), 1 spray in affected nostril bid.
   e. Surgical currettage of the sinus may be necessary if the condition leads to chronic sinusitis and polyp formation.

I. **Infectious mononucleosis**
   1. **History:** Gradual viral infection caused by Epstein-Barr virus (herpesvirus). Usually associated with droplet transmission ("kissing" disease).
   2. **Anatomic location:** Submandibular, occipital, and upper cervical lymphadenopathy.
   3. **Symptoms:** Malaise, fever, sore throat, lymphadenopathy.
   4. **Physical examination:** Tender upper cervical or submandibular nodes. Pharyngitis, tonsillar enlargement, and palatal petechiae may be noted.
   5. **Laboratory findings:**
      a. Atypical lymphocytes in peripheral blood.
      b. Positive Epstein-Barr titer.
      c. Positive Paul-Bunnell test.
      d. Increased serum heterophile level.
      e. Lymphocytosis.
      f. Thrombocytopenia.
      g. Altered liver enzymes (alanine transferase, ALT).
   6. **Treatment:** Symptomatic, including:
      a. Bed rest.
      b. Analgesics.
      c. Antipyretics.
      d. Maintenance of adequate diet and hydration.

III. CYSTIC SWELLING

Swelling caused by cystic enlargement of the face and neck is usually diagnosed by anatomic location and physical examination. These lesions are caused by proliferation of epithelium and formation of a cystic cavity. Occasionally cysts may become secondarily infected and lead to abscess formation and drainage. Characteristics of cystic swellings include:

1. Slow growth.
2. No pain, unless infected.
3. Fluctuance.
4. Found in specific anatomic locations.

Cysts of soft tissues include:

1. Sebaceous cyst
2. Dermoid cyst
3. Thyroglossal duct cyst
4. Branchial cleft cyst
5. Nasoalveolar cyst

A. Sebaceous cyst

Superficial cyst of the skin caused by pilosebaceous dysfunction. These cysts are soft, compressable, and may exhibit a **punctum** (hole) of the overlying skin. The overlying skin is usually adherent to the cyst. These cysts can occur anywhere on the skin.

1. Treatment: Surgical excision.

B. Dermoid cyst

Soft tissue lesion found in the floor of the mouth, with extension into the submental and submandibular regions. Has typical "doughlike" feel and consistency.

1. Treatment: Surgical excision.

C. Thyroglossal duct cyst

Cyst found in the **midline** of the neck, superior to the hyoid bone and inferior to the foramen cecum of the tongue. Usually slow growing and asymptomatic. Moves on swallowing.

1. Treatment: Surgical excision.

D. Branchial cleft cyst (lateral cervical sinus cyst)

Soft tissue enlargement, fluctuant, found in the lateral neck region. Slow growing, circumscribed lesion is found close to the anterior border of the sternocleidomastoid muscle.

1. Treatment: Surgical excision.

E. **Nasoalveolar cyst**
  Soft tissue (fissural) cyst. Found in the lateral aspect of the upper lip beneath the ala of the nose. Lesion is fluctuant and freely moveable.
  1. **Treatment:** Surgical excision.

IV. **SWELLING DUE TO NEOPLASTIC DISEASE**
  Swelling caused by neoplasia of tissue in the face and neck represents tranformation of the tissue. Neoplastic lesions are best diagnosed by symptoms, physical examination, anatomic location, and biopsy. Neoplastic growth can be benign or malignant. Neoplastic lesions may be primary or metastatic to anatomic areas of the face and neck.
  Differential diagnosis is based on:
  1. Anatomic location
  2. Texture and consistency of the swelling
  3. Rate of growth
  4. Circumscribed nature of the swelling
  5. Ulceration
  6. Invasion of vital structures
  7. Dysfunction of anatomic systems
  8. Local and/or systemic symptoms
  Definitive diagnosis is made by histologic evaluation of the lesion by biopsy technique. It is important to correlate the anatomic location of the mass with tissues inherent to the area. This provides a basis for the appropriate workup and diagnosis.
  A. **Diagnosis**
    When a neoplastic growth is suspected, definitive treatment is determined by histologic studies, and clinical and radiographic examinations. Biopsy specimens are used for pathologic examination. Superficial masses and obvious lesions may be totally excised; incisional biopsy is indicated for deeper lesions. Incisional biopsy should not be performed for salivary gland tumors, specifically of the parotid gland (superficial lobe); these tumors can be accurately diagnosed by clinical and radiographic examinations and sialography. Proper surgical technique includes open biopsy, frozen section, and usually superficial lobectomy of the parotid gland.
  B. **Characteristics of neoplastic swelling**
    1. **Benign neoplasms:**
      a. Slow growing.

      b. Low recurrence rate.

      c. Encapsulated.

      d. Freely moveable.

      e. Vital structures displaced.

   2. Malignant neoplasms:

      a. Rapid growth.

      b. High recurrence rate.

      c. Diffuse.

      d. Fixed to tissues.

      e. Vital structures invaded.

C. Treatment

Treatment of neoplastic diseases of the face and neck is based on the histopathologic diagnosis and the clinical presentation of the tumor. Benign tumors are almost always surgically excised. Malignant tumors are staged as to size and the presence or absence of regional or distant metastasis. Treatment methods for malignant tumors include:

  1. Surgery.

  2. Radiation.

  3. Chemotherapy.

V. OBSTRUCTIVE/RETENTIVE SWELLING

Swelling of the face may be caused by blockage of flow of certain physiologic fluids, due to trauma, stricture, or mechanical obstruction (e.g., stone). The two major fluids involved in obstruction are **saliva** and **tears.**

Disorders attributable to obstruction of flow of these fluids include:

  1. Sialadenitis

  2. Sialolithiasis

  3. Ranula

  4. Dacryorhinocystitis

A. Sialadenitis/sialolithiasis

  1. History: Sialadenitis of the major salivary glands is characterized by painful swelling of the affected gland. If the swelling and infection are caused by obstruction, the patient may report intermittent swelling at mealtime. Patients with decreased salivary flow have an increased tendency for sialadenitis. Sialadenitis may also be noted in patients with psychiatric disorders, alcoholism, or xerostomia and in patients with functioning xerostomia secondary to a wide variety of medications, including but not limited to diuretics, tranquilizers, antidepressants, and antihypertensives.

2. **Anatomic location:** Submandibular triangle when infections involve the submandibular gland; preauricular region when swelling involves the parotid gland.

3. **Symptoms:** Swelling of submandibular triangle or preauricular region. May be exacerbated by meals. Erythema may be present over the gland if swelling is severe. The area is usually tender to palpation.

4. **Radiographic/laboratory findings:**
   a. Leukocytosis.
   b. Increased serum amylase level (salivary type).
   c. Salivary stones (sialoliths).

5. **Physical examination:** Swelling of submandibular or preauricular region. May be associated with skin erythema and tenderness. There may be purulent discharge from Stensen's or Wharton's duct.

6. **Treatment:**
   a. Clinical examination and diagnosis.
   b. Occlusal and/or posteroanterior radiographs to rule out sialoliths (stones) of the submandibular or parotid ducts.
   c. Culture and sensitivity testing of any purulent discharge.
   d. Hydration (may require hospital admission and IV fluids).
   e. Palpation and massage of ductal systems.
   f. If stones are absent, dilation of the ducts may be indicated to relieve blockage or to dilate a stricture to facilitate flow or drainage. Dilation is performed using lacrimal probes sizes 0000 to 2.
   g. Broad-spectrum antibiotics
      (1) Dicloxicillin 500 mg PO qid for 7 days.
      (2) Cephalexin (Keflex) 500 mg PO qid for 7 days.

B. **Ranula**

The ranula is a soft tissue lesion in the floor of the mouth that represents a collection of mucus. The lesion may present as facial swelling when it "plunges" through the mylohyoid muscle to the submental or sub-mandibular spaces.

   1. **Treatment:** Surgical excision. May require sublin-gual adenectomy.

C. **Dacryorhinocystitis**

   Dacryorhinocystitis presents as swelling of the superior aspect of the lateral nasal region. It may be soft and fluctuant. The skin may exhibit overlying erythema.

   1. **Treatment:** Surgical excision.

VI. **CONGENITAL/DEVELOPMENTAL SWELLING**

Congenital or developmental lesions that cause changes in the normal anatomy that may be perceived as swelling include **cystic hygroma, masseteric hypertrophy, facial asymmetry,** and **fibrous dysplasia.**

These lesions/conditions have distinct characteristics and are diagnosed by anatomic location, correlation with radiographic changes of the bony skeleton, and concomitant systemic findings.

A. **Cystic hygroma**

   This classic congenital lesion represents a lymphangi-oma in the neck and may appear within the first two decades of life. Treatment is surgical excision.

B. **Masseteric hypertrophy**

   This clinical finding is usually the result of functional muscle hypertrophy as a sequela of parafunctional hab-its. A differentiation can be made by asking patients to clench the jaw and determine if the swelling is related to the muscle. Magnetic resonance imaging can ulti-mately determine the soft tissue cause.

C. **Facial asymmetry**

   Asymmetry of the face can be caused by a variety of factors. Clinical conditions include **facial hemihypertrophy/hemiatrophy, hemifacial microso-mia,** and **condylar hyperplasia.**

   Careful soft and hard tissue analysis must be per-formed. Surgical correction is useful in some cases.

D. **Fibrous dysplasia**

   A disease of unknown cause, fibrous dysplasia may involve bones of the facial skeleton, causing facial swelling and asymmetry. The clinical presentation occurs during the first two decades of life and includes asymmetric facial enlargement of the affected bone. Radiographic findings include radiolucencies and/or radiopacities dependent on the stage of disease. The typical "ground glass" appearance is pathognomonic for the disease. Histologic study allows a definitive diagnosis. Surgical recontouring may be indicated in severe cases.

VII. **TRAUMATIC/POST-SURGICAL SWELLING**

Swelling caused by trauma is related to the location and extent of the traumatic injury. Lacerations, blunt trauma, underlying facial fractures, and other traumatic events will produce **edema** and **hematoma,** manifested as swelling of areas directly related to the traumatic event. In severe trauma the swelling may distort the normal anatomic and geographic structures. With appropriate surgical care, such as repair of fractures and lacerations, the swelling subsides within a few days.

Specific areas of swelling may include temporomandibular joint (TMJ) swelling, which may not be caused by direct trauma but is usually due to forces transmitted through the mandible, causing a hemarthrosis. Symptoms include swelling over the TMJ, limitation of opening, posterior open bite on the affected side, and deviation to the affected side. Treatment includes the use of moist warm compresses, nonsteroidal anti-inflammatory drugs, restriction to a soft diet, and possibly an occlusal splint.

Swelling that occurs after dentoalveolar surgery can be classified as **edema, hematoma,** or **infection.** The differential diagnosis is based on the clinical findings, duration since surgery, and systemic symptoms.

A. **Edema**

Edema is soft, occurs soon after surgery, usually continues for 24 to 36 hours, and begins to decrease in 48 hours.

B. **Hematoma**

A hematoma is a firm mass within the tissues and may be accompanied by ecchymosis. Treatment for a suspected hematoma is application of ice for the first 24 hours, followed by application of moist heat. Antibiotics may be indicated to prevent secondary infection. Aspiration may be performed if the hematoma is superficial.

C. Infection

Postoperative infection usually is manifested by swelling with late onset (>48 hours). Fever and lymphadenopathy are present. Erythema may be present, as well as limitation of function.

BIBLIOGRAPHY

Damion J, Hybels RL: The neck mass: Inflammatory and neoplastic causes. *Postgrad Med* 1987; 81:97–103, 106–107.

Eversole LR: *Clinical Outline of Oral Pathology.* Philadelphia, Lea & Febiger, 1978.

Haddad A, Frenkiel S, Small P: Angioedema of the head and neck. *J Otolaryngol* 1985; 14:14–16.

Shafer WG, Hine MK, Levy BM: *A Textbook of Oral Pathology,* ed 4. Philadelphia, WB Saunders, 1983.

Shugar JM, Som PM, Robbins A, et al: Maxillary sinusitis as a cause of cheek swelling: A rare occurrence. *Arch Otolaryngol* 1982; 108:507–508.

Suckiel JM, Giansanti JB: Cat scratch disease: Report of case and discussion. *J Oral Surg* 1977; 35:54–56.

Topazian RG, Goldberg MH: *Management of Infections of the Oral and Maxillofacial Regions.* Philadelphia, WB Saunders, 1987.

Wood NK, Goaz PW: *Differential Diagnosis of Oral Lesions,* ed 4. St Louis, 1990, Mosby–Year Book.

Oral Mucosal Abnormalities

David A. Lederman

_____

I. Oral mucosal abnormalities
   A. Diffuse gingival erythema
   B. Multifocal erythema of buccal and/or labial mucosa
   C. Focal pigmentation
   D. Multifocal or diffuse pigmentation
   E. Gingival hyperplasia
   F. White lesion of lower lip
   G. Xerostomia
   H. Burning mouth with fibrosis
   I. Atrophic glossitis
   J. Lingual crenation
   K. White lesions of tongue

A diverse group of conditions present as alterations in color, texture, and/or tone of the oral soft tissues. These oral changes may be indicative of local or systemic disease. A rational approach to the differential diagnosis aids in formulating a working or definitive diagnosis and in initiating appropriate therapy.

I. ORAL MUCOSAL ABNORMALITIES
A. Diffuse gingival erythema
A 47-year-old woman has painful gingiva she claims started after a dental prophylaxis 6 months ago. She cannot eat hot or spicy foods or drink alcoholic beverages. The gingiva is sore, and bleeds when she brushes her teeth. Oral hygiene is good. Examination reveals diffuse erythema involving the attached gingiva and alveolar

mucosa, with focal erosions and bleeding points. Involvement of the buccal surfaces is more severe than the lingual and palatal surfaces. Swelling is minimal. Visual evaluation for plaque accumulation and probing of pocket depth reveal minimal periodontal disease, inconsistent with the degree of discomfort or erythema present. No other asymmetries, masses, or lesions are noted in the oral, head, and neck examination. Cursory evaluation of the 12 cranial nerves reveals no abnormalities. Medical and social history are noncontributory, and she takes no medications.

1. **Differential diagnosis:**
   Infection
   Dermatosis
   Nutritional deficiency
   Neoplasia
   Endocrine imbalance
   Allergic reaction

   a. **Infection:** Gingivitis/periodontitis, candidiasis, opportunistic infection, herpes simplex.

      (1) **Gingivitis/periodontitis:** Generalized involvement of both the attached gingiva and the alveolar mucosa in the absence of significant pocket depth or plaque accumulation is inconsistent with common gingivitis or periodontitis.

      (2) **Candidiasis:** Candidiasis and other fungal infections can present as erythematous lesions. While *Candida albicans* is the most common oral fungal infection in humans, other fungi may also infect the oral mucosa. When typical white curdlike colonies are seen elsewhere in the oral cavity, candidiasis is the likely diagnosis. A cytologic smear or a biopsy specimen stained with periodic acid–Schiff stain will demonstrate fungal hyphae and spores if present. *Candida* is a common constituent of the oral flora and usually does not cause infection. When candidiasis is present, therefore, it is appropriate to determine the predisposing

factor or factors. Treatment consists of antifungal medications in the form of rinses, tro-
ches, or pastilles. Side effects are rare. Systemic antifungal medication may be required
for refractory infections but requires monitoring, particularly for alterations in liver enzyme
levels.

(3) **Opportunistic infection** in an immunocompromised host: Immune deficiency may be
hereditary, acquired, or secondary to medication or systemic disease. The most common
infection in the immunocompromised patient is
candidiasis, although a variety of viral, fungal,
bacterial, and parasitic infections have been
reported. A detailed history and physical examination together with appropriate laboratory
studies are necessary for definitive diagnosis.

(4) **Herpes simplex:** Primary herpetic gingivostomatitis often presents with fiery red, painful
gingiva. This acute disease is marked by fever, malaise, regional lymphadenopathy, vesicles, and ulcers. It is seen mainly in children
and young adults, and resolves in 1 to 2
weeks. Treatment is symptomatic and supportive, using topical and systemic analgesics,
fluids, and nutritional supplements. Antibiotics
may be required in patients susceptible to secondary infection. Hospitalization may be necessary for severe cases or for infections in
young children.

b. **Dermatosis:** Pemphigoid, pemphigus, lichen planus, lupus erythematosus.

(1) **Pemphigoid**
Benign mucous membrane pemphigoid is seen
mainly in adults older than 40 years. It is a
vesiculobullous disorder with a marked predilection for the oral mucous membranes. A
desquamative type of gingivitis is a frequent
finding. Ocular involvement is also common.
Scarring lesions of the conjunctiva may result

in blindness. Rubbing unaffected mucosa or skin may result in bulla formation; this is a positive Nikolsky sign and aids in diagnosis. Diagnosis may be made on histologic examination of a biopsy specimen, although special histochemical (immunoperoxidase) stains or immunofluorescence may be necessary to demonstrate antibodies to basement membrane antigens. The patient should be evaluated by his or her physician for extraoral lesions, especially ophthalmic lesions. Mild to moderately severe oral lesions can be managed by topical steroid applications; more severe cases require systemic therapy in cooperation with the treating physician.

Some authors have used the term **gingivosis** to designate desquamative gingivitis occurring in postmenopausal women that is clinically and microscopically similar to benign mucous membrane pemphigoid but without vesicle formation. It persists for 1 to 5 years, then spontaneously resolves.

(2) **Pemphigus vulgaris:** Pemphigus vulgaris is an autoimmune vesiculobullous disease of adults older than 40 years. Oral lesions are usually found, and precede the skin lesions in approximately 50% of all cases. The oral vesicles are more fragile and rupture more readily than those of pemphigoid because they are intraepithelial rather than subepithelial. A positive Nikolsky sign may be elicited. As with benign mucous membrane pemphigoid, the diagnosis of pemphigus vulgaris is made on histologic grounds, possibly requiring immunohistochemical or immunofluorescent techniques to demonstrate antibodies to intercellular antibodies. This disease is chronic, and may be fatal if untreated. Management of pemphigus is by a physician in cooperation with the dental practitioner. Cytotoxic agents or systemic corticosteroids with or without

concomitant azathioprine are used. Oral lesions may be treated with topical steroids with or without concurrent systemic therapy, depending on the severity of the lesions.

(3) **Lichen planus:** Most often lichen planus presents as bilateral, reticular white lesions of the buccal mucosa. Skin lesions are keratotic scales on a purplish background and are found on the extensor surfaces of the wrists and knees. Although lichen planus is classified as a dermatosis, skin lesions need not be present. Erosive lichen planus is a common variant in which erythematous, eroded areas result from cleavage of the epithelium from the underlying connective tissue. Generally, but not universally, the typical white striae are found in some areas of a predominantly erosive case. Lesions most often involve the buccal mucosa, mucobuccal fold, and gingiva. The patient may experience discomfort and/or sensitivity to hot, spicy, or alcoholic foods and beverages. A greater than anticipated incidence of oral carcinomas has been reported in patients with erosive lichen planus. Silverman reported that malignancy developed in 7 (1.2%) of 570 patients. In nonerosive lichen planus diagnosis can usually be made on clinical findings; the erosive type may require biopsy for diagnosis, and more important, to rule out foci of dysplasia or malignant transformation. Patients should be observed and periodic biopsy performed if eroded areas appear to change. Management of symptomatic lichen planus is accomplished with topical steroids, such as fluocinonide (Lidex) 0.05% ointment in Orabase, or betamethasone syrup 0.6 mg/mL. Systemic steroids may be needed initially in severe cases.

(4) **Lupus erythematosus:** Lupus erythematosus is a disorder of unknown cause in which a wide variety of "anti-self" antibodies are pro-

duced. Lesions result from the deposition of antigen-antibody complexes in the tissues. Systemic lupus erythematosus (SLE) has a genetic predisposition. It is seen in females eight times as frequently as in males, and at a younger age, the peak incidence being 30 rather than 40 years, as in males. Diagnosis is based on satisfaction of 4 of 14 clinical and laboratory criteria, one of which is discoid lupus erythematosus (DLE). The prognosis depends on the extent of involvement of the vital organs. Renal and cardiac complications of the immune complex deposits may be life threatening. Urticaria, vesiculation, and maculopapular lesions may occur on the face, trunk, and extremities. The most impressive dermatologic sign is the "butterfly rash" of erythematous lesions across the bridge of the nose and malar areas.

Chronic DLE is a milder form of the disease. It presents as a dermatosis, particularly of the face, scalp, and oral cavity. It is more common than SLE, shares the female predilection, and generally appears in the third or fourth decades of life. Both the chronic discoid (mucocutaneous) and systemic forms are associated with oral lesions. Typical oral lesions have an atrophic center with white dots and a slightly raised border, white radiating striae, and telangiectasia. Erythematous or ulcerative lesions may be seen in SLE as well. Long-standing lesions of several years duration may appear as white plaques. Bilateral involvement of the buccal mucosa is most common, but any intraoral site may be involved. About 6% of patients with DLE eventually develop multisystem manifestations, but many experience complete remission.

(5) **Desquamative gingivitis:** Chronic desquamative gingivitis is the clinical finding in gingival erythema, with separation of the surface epi-

thelium from the underlying connective tissue by light pressure. It is most commonly seen in women older than 40 years; however, both sexes may be affected, at any age.

In a study of 40 patients with desquamative gingivitis, McCarthy et al. diagnosed pemphigoid in 17, pemphigus in 2, and lichen planus in 4; in the remaining 17 patients gingivitis was attributed to hormonal changes, abnormal response to local irritants, and idiopathic factors (Table 8–1). They concluded that desquamative gingivitis was a nonspecific finding that could be attributed to a variety of clinical disorders. In 1976 Rogers et al., using more sophisticated diagnostic methods, found 5 of 7 cases of moderate to severe desquamative gingivitis to be benign mucous membrane pemphigoid.

c. **Nutritional deficiency states:** Vitamin C, vitamin B complex, iron.
Oral mucosal atrophy, glossitis, angular cheilitis, and mucosal ulceration have been associated with deficiencies of iron, folic acid, and vitamin B_{12}. Oral signs and symptoms may appear even before development of anemia. Gingivitis is one of the

TABLE 8– 1.

Desquamative Gingivitis

	McCarthy et al.*		Rogers et al.†	
	n	%	n	%
Benign mucous membrane pemphigoid	17	42.5	5	71.4
Erosive lichen planus	4	10.0	1	14.3
Pemphigus vulgaris	2	5.0		
Hormonal changes	7	17.5		
Irritation	5	12.5		
Idiopathic factors	5	12.5	1	14.3
Total	40	100.0	7	100.0

*Data from McCarthy FP, McCarthy PL, Sklar G: *Oral Surg* 1960; 13:1300–1313.
†Data from Rogers RS, Sheridan PJ, Jordon RE: *Oral Surg* 1976; 42:316–327.

earliest manifestations of vitamin C deficiency, and presents as swelling, bleeding, and ulceration with subsequent loss of osseous support. Deficiency states are discussed further in Case I.

d. **Neoplasia:** Leukemia, erythroplakia/dysplasia, squamous cell carcinoma.

(1) **Leukemia:** Oral pathosis is common in undiagnosed leukemias and frequently contributes to the patient's seeking medical attention. Gingival infiltration by leukemic cells occurs in about half of all patients with acute leukemias. The degree of gingival infiltration and enlargement varies with the type of leukemia, with myelomonocytic and myelocytic types having the highest incidence. The interdental papillae enlarge and may be either hemorrhagic, ulcerated and boggy, or pale and firm. Other signs such as lymphadenopathy, pallor, petechiae and ecchymoses, or malaise are often evident. Complete blood cell count with peripheral smear should be performed. Biopsy may be useful in diagnosis, but should be done with caution because thrombocytopenia can interfere with hemostasis. Treatment of leukemia is the province of the hematologist. When the disease is in remission, routine noninvasive dental treatment may be performed, but the safety of invasive procedures depends on current hematologic profiles. The dentist manages the oral complications of chemotherapy or radiotherapy in cooperation with the hematologist.

(2) **Erythroplakia/dysplasia:** Erythroplakia is a red patch that cannot be clinically diagnosed as another specific entity and which persists after local irritants have been removed. It is usually velvety in texture and may be accompanied by white, leukoplakic areas. The combined red and white lesion is referred to as erythroleukoplakia or simply speckled leukoplakia. Diffuse, focal or multifocal erythro-

plakia is dysplastic (premalignant) or malignant in a large percentage of cases, and should be considered malignant until proved otherwise by biopsy.

(3) **Squamous cell carcinoma:** Multiple sites of oral squamous cell carcinoma may arise by the process of field cancerization. Oral mucosa exposed to promoters and carcinogens, most importantly alcoholic beverages and tobacco, over prolonged periods is at increased risk for carcinoma. Carcinoma diagnosed in one oral site alerts the clinician that other oral sites possibly may demonstrate premalignant changes. Carcinomatous growths may already be demonstrated in these areas, or may develop later. Among patients with oral carcinoma the incidence of multiple cancers of the oral cavity and respiratory and upper gastrointestinal tracts, synchronous or metachronous, has been reported to be as high as 17.7%.

e. **Endocrine imbalance:** Diabetes mellitus, pregnancy, puberty.
Hormonal factors may predispose the patient to an exaggerated periodontal inflammation due to local etiologic agents present in the oral cavity.

f. **Allergic reaction:** Stomatitis venenata/stomatitis medicamentosa.

(1) **Stomatitis venenata/stomatitis medicamentosa:** Allergic mucositis may result from a contact allergen (stomatitis venenata) or from drug hypersensitivity (stomatitis medicamentosa). Any oral site may be involved. Lesions are erythematous and either diffuse or multifocal, sometimes covered by a pseudomembrane, and may be vesicular or ulcerative. Depending on the allergen, lesions may be transient, recurrent, or chronic, and are sometimes accompanied by a burning sensation or pain. Treatment consists of identification and elimination of the allergen. Identification of the

offending agent may require detailed history
and perhaps epimucous patch testing. Acute
reactions are treated with antihistamine and/or
topical corticosteroid therapy.

(2) **Erythema multiforme:** Erythema multiforme
may be idiopathic or associated with either a
viral infection, usually herpesvirus, or a medication, particularly sulfa drugs. In the latter
instance, an allergic basis is accepted. Skin
lesions consist of macules, bullae, and the
classic skin manifestation of erythema multiforme, the target or iris lesion. Intraoral vesicles, erosions, and ulcerations may affect any
site. Painful, crusting, hemorrhagic lesions of
the lips are common. A diagnosis of erythema
multiforme is strongly suggested by rapid-
onset (12–24 hours) target lesions of the skin
and crusting lesions of the lips. Biopsy may
be helpful in confirming the diagnosis and rul-
ing out other vesiculobullous diseases; however, histopathologic findings are not pathognomonic. Stevens-Johnson syndrome is a
severe form of erythema multiforme, involving
the oral cavity, skin, conjunctiva, and genitalia. Young men are most commonly affected.
Depending on severity, treatment of erythema
multiforme consists of antihistamine, corticosteroid, and topical analgesic therapy and
maintenance of nutrition and fluid and electrolyte balance (Table 8–2).

B. **Multifocal erythema**
Routine oral examination of a 58-year-old woman dis-
closed several circinate, erythematous areas on the mandibular labial mucosa and the buccal mucosa bilaterally.
The lesions were 4 to 8 mm in greatest dimension, and
some exhibited a thin white border. The lesions were
asymptomatic, and the patient was unaware of them until
they were brought to her attention. Complete head, neck,
and oral examination revealed no other abnormalities.
Her past medical history was noncontributory, and she
was taking no medications at the time.

TABLE 8–2.

Clinical Comparison of Some Vesiculoulcerative Oral Conditions

Disease	Age at Onset (yr)	Sex	Usual Presentation	Treatment	Prognosis
Dermatosis					
Pemphigoid	>40	M = F	Bullae, ulcers	Steroids	Prolonged course with remissions and exacerbation
Pemphigus	>40	M = F	Bullae, ulcers	Steroids	Prolonged and variable course; may be fatal
Erosive lichen planus	Adult	F > M	Bilateral white intersecting striae with erythematous areas	Steroids	Good
Systemic lupus erythematosus	20–40	F > M	Same as DLE but with vesicles and/or ulcers	Steroids and/or antihistamines and/or antineoplastic agents	Chronic, variable; may be fatal or may diminish over years
Discoid lupus erythematosus	25–45	F > M	"Butterfly rash," red and white lesions, telangiectasis	Steroids and/or antihistamines	Chronic; may diminish over years
Allergy					
Erythema multiforme	Any	M = F	Erythema, vesicles, ulcers	Antihistamines and/or steroids	Good
Erythema multiforme	Young adult	M > F	Rapid onset, target lesions, erythema, crusting lip lesions	Antihistamines and/or steroids	Usually good; may be recurrent

1. **Differential diagnosis**
   Erythema multiforme
   Allergic stomatitis
   Drug reaction
   Erythema migrans
   Lupus erythematosus
   Factitial injury
   Erosive lichen planus
   Candidiasis

   a. **Erythema multiforme:** The term erythema multi-
      forme has been used by some authors to refer to
      chronic, multifocal, nonspecific erythematous le-
      sions of the oral cavity that cannot be classified as
      erythroplakia. We agree with the majority, who
      prefer the more restrictive definition, which in-
      cludes presence of labial or epidermal lesions. For
      a more complete discussion of erythema multi-
      forme, see p. 172.

   b. **Allergic stomatitis:** Allergic stomatitis involving a
      significant portion of the oral mucosa is usually
      symptomatic, but a review of the history for possi-
      ble allergens and observation over 2 to 3 weeks is
      in order. For further discussion see p. 171.

   c. **Drug reaction:** Drug reactions that may or may
      not be due to allergy occasionally manifest on the
      oral mucosa. In addition to irregular erythematous
      or vesicular lesions, mucosal reactions clinically
      and microscopically similar to lichen planus, pem-
      phigoid, or pemphigus have been reported to some
      pharmacologic agents, particularly the thiazides,
      antimalarials, penicillamine, and gold. For further
      discussion see Chapter 13.

   d. **Erythema migrans:** Erythema migrans is also
      known as ectopic geographic tongue, migratory
      stomatitis, erythema circinata, erythema areata
      migrans, and stomatitis areata migrans. Lesions
      may be observed in any oral location, especially
      the buccal and labial mucosae and the floor of the
      mouth. Most often, typical lesions of geographic
      tongue are noted along with the extralingual le-
      sions. Like the lingual counterparts, lesions are

usually multiple, consisting of central atrophic or eroded areas often bordered by a thin, white margin. As one area heals, another undergoes atrophy, giving the illusion that the lesions are migrating. In the absence of lingual lesions, biopsy may be required to establish the diagnosis. Erythema migrans is usually asymptomatic and requires no treatment. Occasionally itching or mild discomfort is reported, which can be alleviated by avoidance of irritating spices and acidic foods and application of topical anesthetics or steroids.

e. **Lupus erythematosus:** Either systemic lupus erythematosus (SLE) or the milder discoid lupus erythematosus (DLE) may produce circinate or discoid oral lesions. The presence of mild oral lesions without concurrent labial or cutaneous lesions militates against this diagnosis; however, Schiodt maintains that oral discoid lesions are not rare, they can be diagnosed in the absence of skin lesions, and such lesions are "not rarely" the first manifestation of SLE or DLE. For further discussion of lupus erythematosus, see p. 167.

f. **Factitial injury:** Self-inflicted trauma may cause white, red, or ulcerated lesions varying from minimal to severe and can cause considerable diagnostic consternation, particularly if the patient in unaware of his or her role in causing the lesions, is incapable of understanding the consequences of his or her habits, or is using the injury as a deviant means of gaining attention or sympathy. The mildest and most common example of factitial injury is cheek chewing, in which an anxious person produces asymptomatic, macerated, shaggy, hyperkeratotic areas, usually bilaterally, on the buccal mucosa. Patients who injure themselves with their fingernails or sharp objects produce single or multiple ulcerations that may become secondarily infected. Those using caustic agents produce chemical burns. Extreme cases of self-mutilation have been reported in psychotic patients and those with certain metabolic disorders (e.g., Lesch-Nyhan syndrome). A thorough history of the lesions should be sufficient for diagnosis in most cases, with follow-up for 1 to 2 weeks to confirm that healing is taking place. Biopsy is indicated if the anticipated resolution does not occur.

g. **Erosive lichen planus:** Typical striae of lichen planus need not be present, and mild erosive forms may be asymptomatic, requiring no treatment. Unless the clinical presentation is typical, however, biopsy is indicated to establish the diagnosis.

h. **Candidiasis:** Candidiasis may have a variety of oral manifestations and may be either symptomatic or asymptomatic. Cytologic smear or histologic study of biopsied tissue, with appropriate instructions to the oral pathologist, will establish the diagnosis.

C. **Focal pigmentation**

A 32-year-old man has been aware of a dark discoloration on the gingiva for several years. The lesion is asymptomatic, and he believes that it has enlarged in the past year. Head, neck, and oral examination yields normal findings except for a solitary 3 by 5 mm bluish black pigmented lesion on the buccal attached gingiva adjacent to the maxillary right first premolar. The border of the discoloration is irregular and fades into the uninvolved mucosa. The tooth is restored with a well contoured, properly fitted ceramometal crown. A periapical radiograph reveals no abnormalities. The patient is taking no medications and has a negative medical history.

1. **Differential diagnosis**

Amalgam tattoo or other foreign body
Nevus
Oral melanotic macule
Melanoma
Benign vascular lesion (varix, hemangioma)
Kaposi's sarcoma

a. **Amalgam tattoo:** Not infrequently, fragments of amalgam are inadvertently introduced submucosally during surgical or restorative procedures.

Amalgam is well tolerated by the tissues, only rarely eliciting significant inflammation or a foreign body reaction. The foreign material appears as an area of localized or somewhat diffuse gray, blue, or black pigmentation. The gingiva is the most frequent site. An appropriately angled radiograph may show radiopaque metallic fragments. Deposits of foreign material that evoke a foreign body reaction may give the clinical impression of slowly spreading as the material is engulfed and dispersed by macrophages. The vast majority of focal pigmented lesions prove to be foreign material, consistent with amalgam tattoo, and require no treatment. However, the possibility of melanoma must be considered. Unless a diagnosis of amalgam tattoo can be made without equivocation, based on radiographic appearance, clinical presentation, or history, biopsy is indicated. The dire consequences of neglecting a malignancy far outweigh the minimal risks of conservative excision.

b. **Nevus:** The nevus, or nevocellular nevus, is a developmental lesion composed of neuroectodermal cells termed nevus cells. It occurs frequently on the skin as a common mole, but occasionally is seen on the oral mucosa. Nevi appear as blue, brown, or black, flat or elevated lesions that do not blanch on pressure, as do vascular lesions. The most common intraoral sites are the hard palate, gingiva, and buccal and labial mucosae. The lesion is removed for histologic study, and no further treatment is necessary.

c. **Oral melanotic macule:** Oral melanotic macule is analogous to ephelis, or freckle, of the skin. It is a flat brown, blue, or black spot resulting from excessive accumulation of melanin in the basal cell layer, the submucosa, or both. The lesion may be clinically indistinguishable from amalgam tattoo, nevus, or early melanoma. It usually presents as a solitary lesion of the vermilion border, gingiva, or buccal mucosa, and occurs twice as frequently in females as in males, and more often in whites than in nonwhites. Biopsy is required to establish a definitive diagnosis.

d. Melanoma: Melanoma is a malignant neoplasm of melanocytes found in the basal cell layer of the epithelium. It is uncommon in the oral cavity, but when found intraorally, the most frequent locations are the palate and the maxillary gingiva and ridge. The average age at onset is about 50 years, and some studies show a nearly 2:1 prevalence in males, whereas other reports show nearly equal sex distribution. Lesions are bluish black or brown, but may be nonpigmented (amelanotic melanoma). Early lesions remain macular for months or years, then become nodular and may ulcerate as they progress. Unlike squamous cell carcinomas, the borders are generally flat and non-indurated. The absence of pain can delay the patient's seeking treatment. Ulceration and bleeding are the most common presenting complaints. Prognosis is strongly influenced by the depth of the tumor, with 0.76 mm a critical landmark. If treated before the nodular stage the prognosis is good. Most cases, however, are not diagnosed early. Metastasis to regional lymph nodes, lung, brain, liver, and bone is common. Treatment is radical surgery, often with postoperative radiation therapy and sometimes with adjuvant chemotherapy or immunotherapy. The 5-year survival rate is less than 15%. The median survival time for oral melanoma is only 18 months after diagnosis, worse than the 67 and 100 months reported for cutaneous melanomas of the head and neck and the trunk, respectively.

e. Benign vascular lesion (varix, hemangioma): A varix is an enlarged, tortuous venule; a hemangioma is a hamartomatous proliferation of blood vessels. Vascular lesions generally appear as raised masses, and may be localized or diffuse. They blanch when compressed. Small lesions may be treated by excision. Large hemangiomas may

be excised, treated by Nd:YAG laser, injected
with sclerosing agents, or left untreated if they do
not interfere with function or appearance.

f. **Kaposi's sarcoma:** Kaposi's sarcoma is a multifocal, mucocutaneous form of angiosarcoma. Since
the early 1980s it has been diagnosed primarily in
patients with acquired immune deficiency syndrome (AIDS), although the classic form of Kaposi's sarcoma occurs mainly in elderly Jewish and
Italian men. In the classic form of the disease lesions are slowly progressive, affecting most often
the lower extremities and seldom causing death. In
patients with AIDS the lesions are rapidly progressive, appearing primarily on the face and neck and
in the oral cavity. Oral lesions are usually multifocal, and may be blue, purple, or brown, presenting as raised plaques or tumor nodules. The most
common intraoral site is the palate. The oral lesions may be excised, cauterized, treated by laser
therapy, or left untreated if they are not hemorrhagic and do not interfere with function. At the
present time AIDS is fatal, usually within 2 to 3
years of diagnosis.

D. Multifocal or diffuse pigmentation

A 26-year-old white man complains of pigmentation of
the oral mucosa. He became aware of the condition 2
months ago and is concerned about it. He admits to having been an intravenous drug abuser, but claims to be
drug free at this time. He takes no medication, but has
smoked three packs of cigarettes daily for 13 years.
Head, neck, and oral examination yield normal findings
except for multiple carious teeth, moderate periodontitis,
and bilateral pigmented lesions of the buccal and labial
mucosae, gingiva, and lateral borders of the tongue. The
lesions are flat, irregular in outline, and vary from light
to dark brown.

1. **Differential diagnosis**

   Physiologic (racial) pigmentation
   Addison's disease
   Neurofibromatosis
   Heavy metal ingestion

Peutz-Jeghers syndrome
Hemochromatosis
Medications
HIV infection

a. **Physiologic pigmentation:** Blacks and dark-skinned nonblacks frequently demonstrate diffuse or multifocal, bilateral pigmentation of the oral mucosa. The gingiva is most often involved, but any oral site may be pigmented. Such pigmentation is present from birth, is normal, and requires no treatment.

b. **Addison's disease:** Primary chronic adrenal cortical insufficiency, or Addison's disease, may result in hyperpigmentation due to increased levels of pituitary melanocyte stimulating hormone. The skin may take on a bronze "tanned" appearance and skin folds appear brown. Pigmentation of the oral mucosa is progressive, bilateral, and either diffuse or multifocal. A history of recent darkening of the pigmentation or systemic manifestations such as weakness, fatigability, hypotension, anorexia, vomiting, diarrhea, or weight loss are suggestive of Addison's disease. Cortisol deficiency also results in the inability to adapt to stress. This presents a potential hazard in certain dental procedures. Evaluation and management by a competent physician is required. Replacement therapy with exogenous corticosteroids generally allows the patient to lead a normal life; however, adjustment of the steroid level at times of stress may be necessary.

c. **Neurofibromatosis:** Neurofibromatosis is a fairly common condition manifesting in childhood. There is no racial or sexual predilection. About half of all cases are inherited by autosomal dominant transmission. The disease is characterized by multiple neurofibromas and pigmented lesions. The neurofibromas are generally cutaneous, but visceral and intraosseous tumors also occur. Cutaneous neurofibromas are either discrete and nodular or diffuse and pendulous. Although the tumors are benign, malignant potential is recognized. Neurofibromatosis has been associated with a variety of malignant tumors, particularly malignant schwannoma. Sarcomas develop eventually in approximately 5% to 15% of patients. The pigmented lesions are variable in size, have smooth borders, and are light brown (café au lait).

d. **Heavy metal ingestion:** Ingestion of certain heavy metals, especially lead, bismuth, and mercury, can cause oral pigmentation. Exposure may be occupational, accidental, or therapeutic. The discoloration is usually seen as a gray border of the marginal gingiva, but may also present as diffuse or discrete pigmentation of the oral mucosa. Ulcerative stomatitis, ptyalism, metallic taste, and swelling of the major salivary glands have also been reported. When present, systemic manifestations of heavy metal toxicity include abdominal pain, anorexia, vomiting, headache, and tremor.

e. **Peutz-Jeghers syndrome:** Peutz-Jeghers syndrome is inherited as an autosomal dominant trait and consists of mucocutaneous pigmentation associated with intestinal polyposis. Distinctive macular melanin deposits are seen on the labial mucosa and the perioral skin as well as the skin around the nostrils and eyes. The buccal mucosa and other intraoral sites may also be involved. Skin lesions on the hands and feet are common. The polyposis involves mainly but not exclusively the small intestine, and patients may experience episodes of abdominal pain, rectal bleeding, or intussusception. Although the polyps themselves do not undergo malignant transformation, malignant tumors of the gastrointestinal tract have been associated with the syndrome. Examination by a gastroenterologist is advisable, but there is no contraindication to dental treatment.

f. **Hemochromatosis:** Hemochromatosis is the excessive deposition of iron pigment within the tissues. The most common form is primary hemosiderosis, an inborn error of metabolism. It is inherited as an autosomal recessive trait affecting predominantly males. Hemochromatosis may also be secondary to alcoholic cirrhosis, thalassemia, portacaval anastomosis, and multiple transfusions, among other factors. Systemic manifestations include diabetes and golden brown pigmentation of the skin. Slate gray to brown pigmentation of the palate and gingiva is due to accumulation of iron and melanin, and may be diffuse or macular. Diagnosis is aided by a history of diabetes and bronze skin along with elevated serum iron concentration.

g. **Medications:** Oral pigmentation due to medications is discussed in Chapter 11.

h. **HIV infection:** A recent article reports 6 cases of sudden onset of pigmented oral mucosal lesions in patients infected with human immune deficiency virus (HIV) type I. In three of the patients pigmentation may be the result of therapeutic and/or recreational drug use, but in three males no known mechanism could be identified.

E. **Gingival hyperplasia**

A 62-year-old woman presents with enlarged, bulbous gingiva. She first noticed the condition 2 months ago, and is concerned because it is cosmetically unattractive and interferes with tooth brushing. The lesions are asymptomatic and more or less symmetric.

1. **Differential diagnosis**

   Gingival fibromatosis

   Leukemic infiltration

   Gingival hyperplasia due to underlying periodontal disease

   Gingival hyperplasia due to medications

   a. **Gingival fibromatosis:** Gingival fibromatosis may be idiopathic or hereditary, inherited as an autosomal dominant trait. It is manifested in early childhood and may interfere with the eruption of the deciduous and permanent teeth. The enlargement occurs primarily in the interdental papillae. It is firm, nontender, and nonhemorrhagic. Hyperplasia is usually self-limiting, but may recur after gingi-voplasty. A familial history and the elimination of other possible causes will establish the diagnosis.

b. **Leukemic infiltration:** For discussion of leukemic infiltration, see p. 170. Diagnosis may be made by gingival biopsy, complete blood cell count, and peripheral smear.

c. **Gingival hyperplasia due to underlying peri-odontal disease:** In the presence of acute inflammation, the diagnosis of periodontal disease is not difficult. Etiologic factors such as plaque, calculus, inadequately restored teeth, and malpositioned teeth are readily apparent. The gingiva is erythematous, edematous, hemorrhagic, and tender. In chronically inflamed gingival tissues, however, these features need not be present; the gingiva is firm, nontender and nonhemorrhagic. Radiographic evidence of periodontitis or a history of periodontal disease or appliance therapy may be helpful. If home care is adequate, gingivoplasty should produce satisfactory results, with no recurrence of the hyperplasia.

d. **Gingival hyperplasia due to medications:** Gingival hyperplasia may occur as a side effect of medications such as phenytoin, nifedipine, and cyclosporin. For further discussion, see Chapter 11.

F. **White lesion of lower lip**

A 73-year-old white man seen on routine examination complains of "stiffness" of his lower lip. Examination shows a diffuse, opaque, white lesion on the vermilion border. Head, neck, and oral examination reveals no other significant findings. He admits to smoking a pipe several hours daily. He takes no medication, and his medical history is noncontributory.

1. **Differential diagnosis**

   Hyperkeratosis/hyperplasia

   Actinic cheilitis

   a. **Hyperkeratosis/hyperplasia:** Epithelial hyperkeratosis or hyperplasia may result from habitual biting or chewing of the lip or from the heat and other irritants associated with pipe, cigar, or cigarette smoking. Diagnosis is made by histologic examination of biopsied tissue.

b. **Actinic cheilitis:** Actinic cheilitis is the result of degenerative changes in the epithelium of the lip due to overexposure to solar or other ultraviolet radiation. Men older than 40 years are most often affected. The most common presentation is that of a diffuse or sharply delineated white surface thickening of the vermilion border of the lower lip. Crusting and/or focal ulceration may be seen. Progression from epithelial hyperplasia or atrophy to dysplasia and carcinoma is common, and biopsy is necessary to determine the extent of cellular changes. Para-aminobenzoic acid (PABA) sunscreen such as PreSun 15 gel is useful in preventing further damage to the lip. Premalignant (dysplastic) actinic cheilitis may be treated topically with 5-fluorouracil cream (Efudex), an antineoplastic antimetabolite. The cream destroys the rapidly dividing dysplastic cells and excoriates the tissue, allowing regeneration. Carcinoma, if present, is treated by surgical excision or radiotherapy. The anticipated 5-year cure rate is better than 80% with either treatment method.

G. **Xerostomia**

A 40-year-old white woman complains that her mouth is sore and that she has difficulty swallowing. She has been aware of this condition for about a year, and thinks it is getting worse. Oral, head, and neck examination reveals xerostomia, generalized atrophy of the oral mucosa, papillary atrophy of the tongue, bilateral angular cheilitis, dry vermilion, and bilaterally enlarged parotid glands. Manipulation of the parotid and submandibular glands produces no secretion from Stensen's or Wharton's ducts. Past medical history and social history are noncontributory. She is a nonsmoker and takes no medication.

1. **Differential diagnosis**
   Medications
   Advanced age
   Depression

Sjögren's syndrome
Mikulicz's disease
Sarcoidosis
Radiation injury
Congenital salivary gland aplasia/hypoplasia
Other systemic disease

a. **Medications:** Numerous pharmacologic agents, including commonly used antihistamines, tranquilizers, and diuretics, can cause xerostomia as an adverse reaction. Drug-induced xerostomia is discussed in Chapter 11.

b. **Advanced age:** Xerostomia secondary to generalized mucosal atrophy is often seen in the elderly as part of the physiologic processes of aging. It may also be seen in women older than 40 years, secondary to endocrine changes in menopause.

c. **Depression:** Depression has long been associated with xerostomia and has been considered by some to be a possible etiologic factor, although a physiologic basis is not clear. We are unaware of any studies assessing salivary flow rates or even of subjective complaints of dryness in clinically depressed patients who are not advanced in age, taking medication, or have some organic systemic disease that itself might cause xerostomia.

d. **Sjögren's syndrome:** The triad of dry eyes, dry mouth, and a connective tissue disease, usually rheumatoid arthritis, constitutes secondary Sjögren's syndrome; in the absence of a connective tissue component the condition is known as primary Sjögren's syndrome (formerly sicca syndrome). Primary Sjögren's syndrome is more likely than secondary to have severe ocular and oral manifestations and carries a higher risk for development of lymphoma. The highest incidence is in women, usually between 40 and 60 years of age. Confirmation of the clinical diagnosis is best made by labial salivary gland biopsy and serum autoantibody assay, particularly for antinuclear antibodies (ANA) and sicca syndrome antibodies A and B (SS-A and SS-B). Sjögren's syndrome is treated by a rheumatologist in cooperation with a dentist, who is primarily responsible for the complications of xerostomia. In most cases Sjögren's syndrome is an uncomfortable but non-life-threatening disease, except for the increased risk of developing lymphomas, up to 40 times the rate for the general population. Therapy is usually conservative and symptomatic. Severe cases may be managed with immunosuppressant drugs. Oral complications of xerostomia are discussed in the following section.

e. **Mikulicz's disease:** Mikulicz's disease is a benign lymphoepithelial lesion of the parotid gland and is related to Sjögren's syndrome. Unlike Sjögren's syndrome, Mikulicz's disease occurs primarily in older men and does not have a connective tissue component. Diagnosis is based on clinical presentation and parotid gland biopsy. Some authors do not accept Mikulicz's disease as a distinct entity, but use the term to denote enlargement of the lacrymal and salivary glands from disorders such as Sjögren's syndrome, sarcoidosis, lymphoma, and leukemia. Oral complications of xerostomia are discussed in the following section.

f. **Sarcoidosis:** Sarcoidosis is a multisystem, noncaseating granulomatous disease that most commonly involves the lungs, lymph nodes, and skin. Involvement of the salivary and lacrymal glands is common, particularly the parotid glands bilaterally. Heerfordt's syndrome and uveoparotid fever are terms used to describe sarcoidosis of the uveal tract and the lacrymal and salivary glands. The cause of sarcoidosis is unknown, but an immunologic mechanism is proposed. It is more common in females than in males, and affects blacks 10 times as often as whites. Patients are usually between 25 and 35 years of age at the time of diagnosis. If the granulomatous infiltration, with its resultant acinar degeneration and fibrosis, involves a significant portion of the glandular tissue, xerostomia will result. Hilar node enlargement, if

present, aids in diagnosis. Positive salivary gland
biopsy or Kveim test are diagnostic. Clinical
course and prognosis are variable from case to
case. Most patients recover with little or no residual impairment. Approximately 10% die of pulmonary fibrosis, cardiomyopathy, or central nervous
system involvement. Oral complications of xerostomia are discussed in the following section.

g. **Radiation injury:** Radiation to the major salivary
glands in excess of 800 cGy causes irreversible
damage, adversely affecting the quantity and
chemical composition of the saliva. The loss of
salivary function may be temporary or permanent,
dependent on the degree of glandular degeneration
and fibrosis. Diagnosis is made from the medical
history. Oral complications of xerostomia are discussed in the following section.

h. **Congenital salivary gland aplasia/hypoplasia:**
Congenital absence or hypoplasia of the major
salivary glands is rare. It may appear either alone
or as part of a syndrome such as an ectodermal
dysplasia. When part of a syndrome, diagnosis is
generally made shortly after birth from the more
significant components of the stigmata.

i. **Other systemic diseases:** Scleroderma and oral
submucous fibrosis are sometimes associated with
xerostomia. In such conditions the dryness of the
mouth is rarely the presenting complaint. Even
less commonly, neurologic disorders affecting salivary gland innervation, vitamin A and B deficiencies, pernicious anemia, Plummer-Vinson syndrome, and diabetes mellitus have also been implicated.

2. **Oral complications of xerostomia**
Oral complications of xerostomia include discomfort,
difficulty in swallowing, accelerated caries rate and
periodontal disease, oral candidiasis, and acute retrograde sialadenitis. Dental caries can be controlled by
reducing dietary sugar, improved home care, applications of fluoride gel in custom trays, and frequent
dental examinations. Prevention of peridontal disease

requires conscientious home care, and may require adjunctive chlorhexidine rinses. Several topical antifungal medications, including nystatin and clotrimazole, are available to treat candidiasis, and systemic antifungal agents such as ketoconazole may be used in refractory cases. However, ketoconazole has been associated with hepatotoxicity and should be used with caution. Acute sialadenitis usually responds to treatment with a penicillinase-resistant penicillin.

H. Burning mouth with fibrosis

A 55-year-old Asian Indian woman complains of "tightness" of the oral mucosa and a burning sensation. Her mouth appears smaller than normal, and the maximum interocclusal distance is limited. Fibrous bands can be palpated in the lips and cheeks. The oral mucosa appears atrophic and is marblelike in color. The remainder of the head, neck, and oral examination yields normal findings. The patient is taking no medication, and the medical history is noncontributory.

1. Differential diagnosis

Oral submucous fibrosis

Scleroderma (progressive systemic sclerosis)

Polymyositis

a. Oral submucous fibrosis: Oral submucous fibrosis is seen primarily in 20- to 40-year-old women of southeast Asia. The cause is uncertain, but irritating spices appear to play a role. The mucosa becomes atrophic and marble-like in appearance due to loss of pigmentation. Patients complain of burning of the mucosa sometimes accompanied by vesicles or ulcerations, either xerostomia or excessive salivation, and altered taste sensation. As the disease progresses the tissues become stiff and fibrotic submucosal bands appear, limiting oral opening and causing difficulty in swallowing. There is no effective treatment. Oral submucous fibrosis is considered premalignant. In one study, 40% of South Indians with oral cancer also had submucous fibrosis.

b. Scleroderma (progressive systemic sclerosis): Scleroderma is a multisystem disorder characterized by vascular changes, fibrosis, and inflammation of the skin and viscera. The cause is unknown, but an autoimmune mechanism is suggested. The age at onset is usually 30 to 50 years, and there is a female predilection estimated to be between 2:1 and 5:1. The hands and face are primarily involved. The skin becomes increasingly stiff and fibrotic and progressively binds to the subcutaneous tissues. Insufficiency of the small blood vessels occurs early in the disease, with prominent telangiectases and frequently Raynaud's phenomenon. The lips become thin and rigid, limiting opening of the mouth. Involvement of the tongue creates difficulty in masticating, swallowing, and speaking. Xerostomia is a frequent finding and in some cases is related to coexisting Sjögren's syndrome. Widening of the periodontal ligament space on dental radiographs is a characteristic finding, and areas of resorption may be seen on the inferior border of the mandible, the ramus, the condyles, and/or the coronoid process. Exposure of the teeth due to involvement of the facial skin predisposes the patient to caries and periodontal disease, whereas immobile oral mucosa is prone to trauma from food or prosthetic appliances. Proper oral hygiene may be difficult or impossible, especially in the posterior areas, and otherwise restorable teeth may require extraction because of limited access by the patient and the dentist. There is no effective treatment for progressive systemic sclerosis. It generally progresses until death intervenes, usually due to renal, cardiac, or respiratory failure or to intestinal malabsorption.

c. **Polymyositis:** Dermatomyositis or polymyositis is a disorder of unknown cause related to systemic sclerosis. The clinical history may include edema, dermatitis, myositis, neuritis, mucositis, and calcinosis. Onset is usually in the sixth decade, but patients of any age may be affected. The disease may be acute or chronic. Oral manifestations include stomatitis, pharyngitis, telangiectasis, and involvement of the oral and facial muscles leading to constriction of the labial orifice, palpable fibrous bands, and soft tissue calcifications. There is no specific treatment for polymyositis, although steroid therapy has been beneficial. The prognosis is variable: some patients have only mild disability; others die of the disease or from visceral malignancies, which are reported in as many as 20% of patients.

I. Atrophic glossitis

A 74-year-old woman complains of painful mouth of 3 months duration. She states that her tongue is sore and that she cannot eat or drink anything hot or spicy. Her tongue is devoid of filiform papillae, but some fungiform papillae remain. Salivary flow and consistency are clinically normal. The skin and oral mucosa are somewhat pale, and she admits to tiring easily on exertion. Head, neck, and oral examination yield normal findings, and the medical history is noncontributory.

1. Differential diagnosis

Pernicious anemia
Iron deficiency
Folic acid deficiency
Vitamin B complex deficiency
Radiation/chemotherapy
Allergic stomatitis

a. Pernicious anemia: In pernicious anemia, there is a deficiency of intrinsic factor, a mucoprotein produced by the gastric parietal cells that is required for absorption of vitamin B_{12} across the ileum. The deficiency is believed to have an autoimmune basis, and 20% of patients have a family history of the disorder. It occurs late in life, hardly ever before the age of 35 years. Males and females are equally affected. Signs and symptoms include pallor, fatigability, shortness of breath, atrophic glossitis, and progressive peripheral neuritis. Peripheral blood and marrow specimens show a macrocytic anemia, with abnormally shaped erythrocytes, platelets, and neutrophils. If untreated, progressive degeneration of the spinal cord leads to paresthesias of the extremities, incoordination, and weakness. Early treatment with parenteral vitamin B_{12} may prevent the neurologic symptoms. Steroids can reverse the hematologic abnormalities, allow regeneration of the gastric mucosa, and improve intrinsic factor levels.

b. **Iron deficiency:** The most common anemia is that due to iron deficiency. Estimates of iron deficiency in U.S. women range from 5% to 30%, due to menstrual blood loss. In males the most common cause is bleeding peptic ulcer. Atrophic glossitis and angular cheilitis may be seen in iron deficiency states before other manifestations of the anemia. The glossitis is not so severe as in folate or vitamin B_{12} deficiency. Treatment consists of determining the underlying cause and correcting it if appropriate. Iron supplements may be prescribed for women with clinically significant physiologic blood loss.

c. **Folic acid deficiency:** Folates are found in most raw vegetables and fruits, although cooking depletes them. Deficiency of folic acid is seen mainly in patients with inadequate diet, particularly those with increased vitamin demand as in pregnancy. To a lesser extent, patients with malabsorption syndromes may also have folic acid deficiency. Hematologic findings mimic those described for pernicious anemia, but the neurologic changes are absent. Atrophic glossitis and angular cheilitis are often seen, and in severe cases ulcerative mucositis and pharyngitis. Diagnosis is based on hematologic findings along with normal serum vitamin B_{12} and low serum folic acid levels. Treatment consists of oral vitamin supplements. Of interest, some antineoplastic chemotherapeutic agents are folic acid antagonists and induce hematologic changes and mucosal lesions of folic acid deficiency.

d. **Vitamin B complex deficiency:** Deficiency of one or more of the B vitamins may cause mucosal atrophy, papillary atrophy of the tongue, and angular cheilitis. Diagnosis may be made by serum analysis for the individual vitamins, but this is an unnecessary and expensive procedure because deficiencies are usually multiple, the disorder is seldom a serious health threat, and the treatment is combined supplements of the B complex vitamins. If the differential diagnosis can be narrowed to vitamin B complex deficiency, empirical treatment may be justified, and the results monitored at monthly intervals.

e. **Radiation/chemotherapy:** Radiation to the oral cavity and/or chemotherapy may be determined by history. Oral complications of radiation to the head and neck include mucositis, xerostomia, secondary infections, sensitivity of teeth, impaired taste sensation, muscle trismus, and osteoradionecrosis. Complications of chemotherapy include mucositis, xerostomia, neurotoxicity, and bone marrow suppression, which predisposes the patient to infection and excessive bleeding. Management of these oral complications is discussed in Chapter 10.

f. **Allergic stomatitis:** See discussion, p. 171.

2. **Management of atrophic glossitis**

Complete blood count with differential and peripheral smear, iron, ferritin, folic acid and vitamin B_{12} should be performed. Vitamin B_{12} deficiency, especially in the presence of megaloblastic anemia, should be managed by a physician.

J. **Lingual crenation**

A partially edentulous 48-year-old male stockbroker has a slightly enlarged tongue with a scalloped border. The indentations correspond with the outlines of the lingual surfaces of the remaining mandibular teeth. Wear facets are noted on the occlusal surfaces of many teeth, and he admits to nocturnal bruxism. The temporomandibular joint, the orofacial musculature, and the 12 cranial nerves appear to be functioning within physiologic limits. No other abnormalities of the head, neck, or oral cavity are observed or reported. He was unaware of the condition of his tongue until it was brought to his attention by his dentist. Medical history is noncontributory.

1. **Differential diagnosis**

   Habit pattern

   Lingual edema

   Loss of muscle tone/enlargement of tongue

   Tumor

   a. **Habit pattern:** Pressing the tongue against the teeth as a habit or as a reaction to stress may be difficult to document because the patient generally is unaware of it. Once advised that lingual disfigurement could be self-inflicted, the patient may interrupt and eventually break the habit or may accept it as innocuous. In this case, no treatment is necessary. Deviant swallowing habits in children not only may cause lingual crenation but may cause or perpetuate malocclusion. Appliance therapy and/or speech therapy are usually required to establish an adult swallowing pattern.

   b. **Lingual edema:** Edema of the tongue may be associated with acute stomatitis, for example, acute necrotizing gingivostomatitis, primary herpetic gingivostomatitis, or erythema multiforme, but is not the prominent feature of these diseases. The typical lesions of acute necrotizing ulcerative gingivitis or the herpetic vesicles and ulcers confirm these diagnoses. Fever and malaise are commonly noted as well. Similarly, erythema multiforme sufficiently severe to cause noticeable lingual edema would present with extralingual lesions, particularly hemorrhagic and crusting lesions of the lips.

   c. **Loss of muscle tone/enlargement of the tongue** may be associated with Down syndrome and with certain endocrine disturbances, particularly myxedema, Cushing's syndrome, acromegaly, gigantism, and congenital hypothyroidism. All are associated with significant, easily visualized alterations in facial features or stature that facilitate diagnosis.

   d. **Tumor:** Slow growing masses of the tongue, neoplastic and nonneoplastic, such as granular cell tu-

tumors, neurofibromas, lymphangiomas, hemangiomas, and amyloidosis, may cause macroglossia, either primarily or secondarily, by blockage of efferent lymphatic vessels. Palpation of the tongue will disclose a submucosal mass. Diagnosis must be made by histologic examination of biopsy tissue.

K. **White lesions of tongue**

A 24-year-old male student is seen on routine dental recall. Oral examination reveals bilateral asymptomatic white lesions of the lateral borders of the tongue. The lesions have a somewhat shaggy texture. Results of head, neck, and oral examination are otherwise within normal limits. Medical history is noncontributory. On questioning, the patient admitted to homosexual relationships.

1. **Differential diagnosis**

Epithelial hyperplasia/hyperkeratosis
Candidiasis
Hairy leukoplakia

a. **Epithelial hyperplasia/hyperkeratosis:** White patches due to epithelial hyperplasia and/or hyperkeratosis are not uncommon, especially on the lateral borders of the tongue. Such lesions generally result from mild trauma such as from chewing the tongue or from sharp or irregular surfaces of teeth, restorations, or appliances. The lesions resolve when the irritating factor is corrected. No further treatment is required.

b. **Candidiasis:** Candidiasis is discussed earlier in this chapter. Hyperplastic white lesions are a frequent finding, and appropriately stained cytologic smears or biopsy specimens will demonstrate the fungal organisms. It should be borne in mind, however, that candidal colonization does not always imply candidal cause. In certain instances the fungi may colonize another more significant lesion. If a smear is positive for fungi but the lesion does not respond to antifungal therapy, biopsy is required.

c. **Hairy leukoplakia:** Hairy leukoplakia presents as white lesions that do not rub off and which have a corrugated, shaggy, or hairlike texture. It is seen primarily on the tongue, usually bilaterally, and most often on the lateral borders, but has also been reported on the buccal and labial mucosa, the floor of the mouth, the palate, and the oropharynx. Biopsy is required for diagnosis. Approximately 50% of patients are secondarily infected by *Candida*. Immunohistochemical staining demonstrates Epstein-Barr virus (EBV) within epithelial cells, and Sciubba has suggested that hairy leukoplakia is an opportunistic infection by EBV in immunocompromised patients. EBV is part of the normal oral milieu in many patients, as evidenced by the high incidence of anti-EBV antibodies in the sera of healthy adults. Hairy leukoplakia is a fairly reliable marker for human immunodeficiency virus (HIV) infection, especially when diagnosed in patients at high risk for acquired immune deficiency syndrome (AIDS). Cases have been reported, however, of lesions clinically and microscopically identical to those of hairy leukoplakia in non–high risk patients who prove HIV-negative. Green and co-workers proposed the term "pseudo–hairy leukoplakia" for these lesions.

BIBLIOGRAPHY

Lichen planus
   Silverman S (ed): *Oral Cancer,* ed 2. New York, American Cancer Society, 1985, p 27.

Lupus erythematosus
   Gilliam JN, Sontheimer RD: Skin manifestations of SLE. *Clin Rheum Dis* 1982; 8:207.
   Schiodt M: Oral manifestations of lupus erythematosus. *Int J Oral Surg* 1984; 13:101–147.

Leukemia
   Hou G-L, Tsai C-C: Primary gingival enlargement as a diagnostic indicator in acute myelomonocytic leukemia. *J Periodont* 1988; 59:852–855.
   Stafford R, Sonis S, Lockhart P, et al: Oral pathoses as diagnostic indicators in leukemia. *Oral Surg* 1980; 50:134–139.

Erythroplakia
   Gluckman JL, Crissman JD, Donegan JO: Multicentric squamous
   cell carcinomas of the upper aerodigestive tract. *Head Neck Surg*
   1980; 3:90–96.
   Mashberg A: Erythroplasia: The earliest sign of asymptomatic
   oral cancer. *J Am Dent Assoc* 1978; 96:615–620.
   Waldron CA, Shafer WG: Leukoplakia revisited: A clinicopathologic study of 3,256 oral leukoplakias. *Cancer* 1975; 36:1386–
   1392.

Allergic reaction
   Eversole LR: Allergic stomatitides. *J Oral Med* 1979; 34:93–
   102.

Erythema migrans
   Littner MM, Dayan D, Gorsky M, et al: Migratory stomatitis.
   Oral Surg 1987; 63:555–559.

Factitial injury
   Altom RL, DiAngelis AJ: Multiple autoextractions: Oral self-
   mutilation reviewed. *Oral Surg* 1989; 67:271–274.
   Fusco MA, Freedman PD, Black SM, et al: Munchausen's syndrome: Report of case. *J Am Dent Assoc* 1986; 112:210–212.

Nevus
   Buchner A, Hansen LS: Pigmented nevi of the oral mucosa: A
   clinicopathological study of 32 new cases and review of 75 cases
   from the literature. Part I. *Oral Surg* 1979; 48:131–142.

Oral melanotic macule
   Buchner A, Hansen LS: Melanotic macule of the oral mucosa: A
   clinicopathologic study of 105 cases. *Oral Surg* 1979; 48:244–
   249.

Melanoma
   Gussack GS, Fisher SR: Cutaneous melanoma of the head and
   neck. *Arch Otolaryngol* 1983; 109:803–808.

Neurofibromatosis
   D'Agostino AN, Soule EH, Miller RH: Sarcomas of the peripheral nerves and somatic soft tissues associated with multiple neurofibromatosis (von Recklinghausen's disease). *Cancer* 1963;
   16:1015–1027.

HIV infection
   Langford A, Pohle HD, Gelderblom H, et al: Oral hyperpigmentation in HIV-infected patients. *Oral Surg* 1989; 67:301–307.

Actinic cheilitis
  Payne TF: An evaluation of actinic blocking agents for the protection of lip mucosa. *J Am Dent Assoc* 1976; 92:409–411.
  Warnock GR, Fuller RP Jr, Pelleu GB: Evaluation of 5-fluorouracil in the treatment of actinic keratosis of the lip. *Oral Surg* 1981; 52:501–505.

Xerostomia
  Mahvash N, Ship II: Xerostomia: Diagnosis and treatment. *Am J Otolaryngol* 1983; 4:283–292.

Sjögren's syndrome
  Scully C: Sjögren's syndrome: Clinical and laboratory features, immunopathogenesis and management. *Oral Surg* 1986; 62:510–523.

Mikulicz's disease
  Robbins SL, Cotran RS, Kumar V: *Pathologic Basis of Disease,* ed 3. Philadelphia, WB Saunders, 1984, p 190.

Salivary gland hypoplasia
  Bartlett RD, Eversole LR, Adkins RS: Autosomal recessive hypohydrotic ectodermal dysplasia: Dental manifestations. *Oral Surg* 1972; 33:736–742.

Oral submucous fibrosis
  Pindborg JJ, Zachariah J: Frequency of oral submucous fibrosis among 100 South Indians with oral cancer. *Bull WHO* 1965; 32:750–753.

Polymyositis
  Sanger RG, Kirby JW: The oral and facial manifestations of dermatomyositis with calcinosis. *Oral Surg* 1973; 35:476–488.

Hairy Leukoplakia
  Sciubba J, Brandsma J, Schwartz M, et al: Hairy leukoplakia: An AIDS-associated opportunistic infection. *Oral Surg* 1989; 67:404–410.
  Green TL, Greenspan JS, Greenspan D, et al: Oral lesions mimicking hairy leukoplakia. *Oral Surg* 1989; 67:422–426.

Early Oral Squamous Carcinoma

Arthur Mashberg

_____

Approximately 29,000 new cases of oral and oropharyngeal cancers (primarily squamous) are documented each year in the United States. If we include other squamous aerodigestive cancers (lung, larynx, esophagus, hypopharynx) that have a common cause (cigarette smoking and alcohol consumption) and frequently coexist as second primary cancers, we can add another 175,000 cases of squamous cancers yearly. An early diagnosed oral cancer may be used as a "flag" to identify those patients at high risk for these cancers.

It is generally accepted that stage more than any other factor influences the duration of survival and that oral cancers less than 1 cm in diameter should be as curable as early observed skin cancers. Size and symptoms are related, and although the oral cavity is easily accessible for visual examination, early cancers are often not diagnosed when they are asymptomatic. Generally at time of diagnosis most lesions are large and symptomatic, with at least 50% of patients demonstrating cervical lymph node metastasis. These lesions usually demonstrate induration, ulceration, and bleeding—the so-called classic signs of cancer. Although in recent years surgery, radiation therapy, and chemotherapy have improved the quality of survival after treatment, the overall 5-year survival rate remains 40% to 50%.

Primary prevention of oral and oropharyngeal squamous cancer by eliminating etiologic or risk factors has not occurred. Secondary prevention, by virtue of early recognition and treatment, is available and feasible.

Squamous cancer is favorable for early diagnosis because it affects predominantly an identifiable risk group (heavy drinkers and smokers) and has a fairly lengthy and detectable asymptomatic phase. In addition there is a well-developed technical screening method (toluidine blue application and/or rinse) for its identification. After biopsy, treatment of early squamous cell carcinoma may be accomplished by wide local excision, with minimal deformity, and in some instances by radiotherapy.

I. RISK FACTORS

Cigarette smoking in combination with alcohol ingestion has been identified in the United States and Western Europe as the prime and most significant risk factor in the development of oral and oropharyngeal cancer. A number of epidemiologic studies show conclusively that the risk for a person who smokes one pack of cigarettes a day is approximately four times that of nonsmokers, whereas the risk to that same smoker who is also a heavy drinker is about 15 times. Experimentally, combustion products of tobacco have been shown to be carcinogenic, whereas there is no conclusive experimental evidence to suggest the same for alcohol. It is believed that alcohol may affect the patient's immune competence and thereby permit cancers to thrive and grow. However the direct contact effect of alcohol cannot be excluded.

In the US culture, pipe and cigar smoking is identified as a risk factor, although such habit is minimal compared with the cigarette-alcohol habit. Smokeless tobacco has been indicated as a risk factor, primarily related to verrucous carcinoma, a highly differentiated variant of squamous cancer, with limited incidence in the United States.

In the past, chronic irritation, broken down and sharp cusps, hot and spicy foods, chemical agents, and denture irritation, among other factors, were suggested as etiologic agents for the development of oral malignancies. The evidence suggests that physical irritation is not a significant factor. It has been found that the most traumatized areas of the oral cavity (hard palate, alveolus, cheeks) have the lowest incidence of cancers. The past relationships between syphilis and vitamin deficiencies and cancer have been essentially discredited by present knowledge. There are suggestions that lichen planus may develop into oral cancer in less than 1% of patients. This is highly conjectural, with no solid evidence to support this concept.

II. HIGH-RISK INTRAORAL SITES

There are distinct cultural and geographic differences in the distribution of cancers within the oral cavity. Cancers related to cigarettes and alcohol consumption, habits that predominate in the United States and Western Europe, are found primarily in the floor of the mouth, mid and posterior ventrolateral tongue, and soft palate complex, which comprises the uvula, soft palate, anterior tonsillar pillars, and the lingual aspect of the retromolar trigone. Occurrence in these anatomic locations may be related to the diffusion of cigarette smoke into these areas by the action of the tongue, cheeks, and soft palate rather than by direct contact with the cigarette. The cancers found in these areas are usually erythroplastic (red and inflamed), with minimal keratinization. "Leukoplakic," or highly keratinized, cancers do not commonly occur in these sites in this population.

Lesions found in pipe or cigar smokers are usually in the buccal areas and lateral aspects of the tongue, sites where the tip of the pipe stem or the end of the cigar are in direct or close contact with the mucous membrane, presumably allowing concentrated streams of smoke to create a carcinogenic effect. These lesions are usually more highly keratinized than the alcohol-cigarette cancers and have a much lower incidence. Verrucous carcinoma is frequently found at the site of placement of the unburned smokeless tobacco, and is keratinized.

In India, where oral cancer is a major health problem and the most predominant form of squamous cancer, it appears that the common habit of placing a quid composed of betel nut, tobacco, and often lime in the buccal pouch or sulcus is the etiologic agent. These cancers develop at the site of placement and are usually well differentiated.

III. CLINICAL EXAMINATION OF INTRAORAL SITES

The high-risk sites require careful scrutiny in an effective oncologic examination of the oral cavity. These areas are difficult to evaluate without adequate lighting. Standard dental lights and some fiber optic light systems appear to be best for detection of early lesions. Head mirrors and lamps do not have sufficient intensity or color balance to allow an appreciation of minute mucosal alterations, especially erythroplastic inflamed areas.

A dental or laryngeal mirror facilitates adequate visualization of areas that cannot be seen directly. Use of a tongue depressor as a retractor does not permit visualization of all significant intraoral mucosal surfaces, because light cannot be directed or reflected with the instrument. The mouth mirror is more rigid and better tolerated by patients.

For evaluation of the anterior and middle thirds of the floor of the mouth and the anteroventral two thirds of the tongue, the mandible should be horizontal when the mouth is open. The tip of the tongue should be extended upward, contacting the hard palate posteriorly. This maneuver will expose the site of most frequent occurrence, especially the papilla at the exit of Wharton's duct. Indirect mirror examination of the lingual aspect of the anterior alveolus may be necessary.

Examination of the posterior floor of the mouth, retromolar trigone, and posterior ventrolateral aspect of the tongue (including the area of the foliate papillae) necessitates grasping the anterior third of the tongue with a gauze sponge, distracting it to the contralateral labial commissure, and withdrawing it from the oral cavity as far as possible. External pressure in the area of the submandibular gland on the ipsilateral side permits the posterior floor of the mouth to be elevated and its contiguous structures to be visualized. At the same time, the mirror should be used to view, indirectly, the lingual aspect of the retromolar trigone. With the tongue still hyperextended, the anterior tonsillar pillar (glossopalatine fold) may also be evaluated. The soft palate, uvula, and posterior pillars may be visualized directly by depressing the middle third of the tongue and having the patient inhale deeply.

Although palpation is an important part of head and neck examination, direct visualization of mucosal surfaces is more significant in detecting early lesions, which usually have little mass and minimal depth. Mirror examination should be used for lesions in the base of the tongue and vallecula, because these areas are not accessible for direct visualization.

Clinical Appearance

Symptomatic Cancer

Cancer of the oral cavity and oropharynx assumes many different appearances during its progression from a minimal or non-visual clinical lesion to a symptomatic lesion. By the time a carcinoma becomes symptomatic, producing pain or dysfunction, it usually is 1 to 2 cm in diameter, and frequently is larger. It is not uncommon for the patient to be comparatively comfortable, with minimal dysfunction, until the lesion is 3 to 4 cm in diameter and has invaded deeper structures, such as muscles of the tongue and muscles of mastication and/or the mandible.

Symptomatic lesions generally reveal some, if not all, of the following characteristics: induration, exophytic growth, ulceration, multiple surface changes including granularity, occasional bleeding, keratin formation, inflammation, and interference with function. Invasion of bony structures may be seen on radiographs. At least 50% of these patients have concomitant cervical lymphadenopathy, usually submandibular or jugulodigastric, due to metastasis.

These lesions and their sequelae can be considered late in the course of the cancer. It is well established that cancer, after its initiation, may persist for a considerable period before producing symptoms. There is an apparent long asymptomatic phase during which the cancer enlarges. Therefore it behooves the clinician to develop a set of criteria by which to diagnose early asymptomatic cancer that displays none or few of the above-mentioned signs and symptoms.

IV. CLINICAL EXAMINATION OF NECK FOR LYMPHADENOPATHY

An oral and oropharyngeal cancer examination must include careful evaluation of the lymph node groups of the neck to which head and neck cancers may metastasize. This examination should be accomplished prior to any biopsy procedure, because post-biopsy examination may reveal nodes that are related to the procedure rather than to the suspect lesion.

Specific lymph node groups are significant. Most oral cancers metastasize to the submandibular nodes lying between the skin and the submandibular salivary gland. These are palpable approximately one to two fingerbreadths below the inferior border of the mandible at approximately the level of the mandibular notch. Palpation should be accomplished by external examination, palpating the area through the skin, and via bidigital palpation, placing one finger into the floor of the mouth and the other externally to allow for discernment of submandibular nodes lying on the submandibular gland.

The next group of lymph nodes evaluated are the deep cervical nodes located under the anterior border of the sternomastoid muscle, in the anterior triangle, extending from the angle of mandible to the clavicle. These may be termed the superior, middle, and inferior deep cervical nodes. Of most significance in metastasis of posterior oral cavity and oropharyngeal cancers are the superior deep cervical nodes, or jugulodigastric nodes. The inferior deep cervical nodes when they are related to lung metastasis are called supraclavicular nodes, located above the clavicle at the posterior edge of the inferior portion of the sternomastoid muscle at its attachment to the clavicle. All node groups are interrelated! Occasionally oral cancers may metastasize, unexpectedly, to lower nodes in the neck.

Palpation of nodes is accomplished with minimal pressure so that small nodes are not compressed and overlooked. Palpation should be accomplished with the patient's head tilted toward the ipsilateral side of the neck being examined, to decrease muscle tension that may obscure small nodes. Collapsing the patient's neck to the ipsilateral side reduces fascial tension and permits finger exploration beneath the sternomastoid muscle. The carotid sinus and hyoid bone may be confused with nodes. The pulsations of the carotid and movement of the hyoid on swallowing rule out the possibility of these structures being confused with nodes.

Positive findings should be correlated with the presence of lesions in the oral cavity and oropharynx. Obvious neck nodes that have no associated oral or oropharyngeal lesions should be considered suspect and possibly related to lesions of the hypopharynx or larynx.

V. ASYMPTOMATIC EARLY CANCER/ ERYTHROPLASIA

Asymptomatic cancers in western cultures, where cigarette smoking and alcohol consumption predominate as risk factors, often appear as erythroplastic changes, with some mucosal atrophy, in high risk sites. These lesions may be 2 to 3 mm to 2 to 3 cm in diameter, yet remain asymptomatic because of minimal invasion. Penetration beyond the basement membrane is still limited. A host response that results in an inflammatory barrier below the invasive tumor imparts a clinical appearance of redness or erythroplasia. This response appears clinically as inflammation, not a plaque!

These early erythroplastic lesions have two distinct clinical appearances: The first is a granular, red, velvety lesion, with or without stippled or patchy areas of keratin lying within or peripheral to the lesion. The keratinized areas appear to be lying on an inflamed mucosal surface that may appear atrophic and worn. Their appearance can be compared with areas of worn fabric with a granular surface. The other common appearance is a smooth, nongranular area, primarily red, with minimal or no keratin evident. Few of these lesions are elevated, palpable, bleeding, or ulcerated. Rarely is cervical metastasis present at this stage.

These changes in the mucosal surface may not have well-defined boundaries. They may blend irregularly with normal mucosa, and frequently there appear to be islands of entrapped normal mucosa within the red, inflamed areas. On occasion there may be a second or third lesion in areas adjacent to or at a distance from the first noted lesion, due to field cancerization.

Because these cancers may simulate nonspecific inflammatory conditions, the most effective method of reducing the number of excessive biopsies is to allow a 10- to 14-day interval with withdrawal of all possible sources of inflammation (e.g., chronic trauma related to dentures, hot and spicy foods) prior to determination of biopsy site. In addition, pathologic entities such as moniliasis and erythema multiforme should be ruled out. If the lesion is still present at the second visit, biopsy is mandatory.

Keratin or leukoplakia may or may not be present and is not diagnostic. More highly diagnostic is persistent erythroplasia; clinicopathologic studies support the essential congruity between erythroplakia and carcinoma. It should be noted that carcinoma in situ does not appear clinically different from early carcinoma; both usually appear erythroplastic.

VI. CLINICAL DOCUMENTATION

Lesions clinically suspect for cancer should be documented properly prior to biopsy, with notation of location, size, surface texture, and elevation (in millimeters), and presence of ulceration, bleeding, induration, and cervical lymphadenopathy; in addition, clinical staging should be accomplished (Figs 9–1 and 9–2).

VII. BIOPSY AND DIAGNOSTIC AIDS

A persistent lesion should be biopsied regardless of clinical suspicion, unless the clinician is absolutely certain, without qualification, that the lesion is benign. Incisional biopsy is preferred to establish a diagnosis. Excisional biopsy of suspected cancers is not appropriate, because tissue must be excised to a minimum of 1 cm in all directions, including depth. Excisional biopsy results in scar contracture and deformity within the oral cavity, and may add to confusion regarding exact location and

Data Form for Cancer Staging

Patient identification

Name _____

Address _____

Hospital or clinic number _____

Age ____ Sex ____ Race _____

Oncology Record

Anatomic site of cancer _____

Histologic type _____

Grade (G) _____

Date of classification _____

Institution identification

Hospital or clinic _____

Address _____

Chronology of classification

(use separate form for each time staged)

[ ] Clinical (use all data prior to first treatment)

[ ] Pathologic (if definitively resected specimen available)

Stage Grouping

[ ] 0	Tis	N0	M0
[ ] I	T1	N0	M0
[ ] II	T2	N0	M0
[ ] III	T3	N0	M0
	T1	N1	M0
	T2	N1	M0
	T3	N1	M0
[ ] IV	T4	N0	M0
	T4	N1	M0
	Any T	N2	M0
	Any T	N3	M0
	Any T	Any N	M1

Definitions

Primary Tumor (T)

[ ] TX Primary tumor cannot be assessed

[ ] T0 No evidence of primary tumor

[ ] Tis Carcinoma in situ

[ ] T1 Tumor 2 cm or less in greatest dimension

[ ] T2 Tumor more than 2 cm but not more than 4 cm in greatest dimesion

[ ] T3 Tumor more than 4 cm in greatest dimension

[ ] T4 (Lip) Tumor invades adjacent structures, e.g., through cortical bone, tongue, skin of neck

[ ] T4 (Oral cavity) Tumor invades adjacent structures, eg., through cortical bone, into deep (extrinsic) muscle of tongue, maxillary sinus, skin

Lymph Node (N)

[ ] NX Regional lymph nodes cannot be assessed

[ ] N0 No regional lymph node metastasis

[ ] N1 Metastasis in a single ipsilateral lymph node, 3 cm or less in greatest dimension

[ ] N2 Metastasis in a single ipsilateral lymph node, more than 3 cm but not more than 6 cm in greatest dimension; or multiple ipsilateral lymph nodes, none more than 6 cm in greatest dimension; or bilateral or contralateral lymph nodes, none more than 6 cm in greatest dimension

[ ] N2a Metastasis in a single ipsilateral lymph node more than 3 cm but not more than 6 cm in greatest dimension

[ ] N2b Metastasis in multiple ipsilateral lymph nodes, none more than 6 cm in greatest dimension

[ ] N2c Metastasis in bilateral or contralateral lymph nodes, none more than 6 cm in greatest dimension

[ ] N3 Metastasis in a lymph node more than 6 cm in greatest dimension

Distant Metastasis (M)

[ ] MX Presence of distant metastasis cannot be assessed

[ ] M0 No distant metastasis

[ ] M1 Distant metastasis

Location of Tumor

[ ] Lips; Upper
Lower

[ ] Buccal mucosa

[ ] Floor of mouth

[ ] Oral tongue

[ ] Hard palate

[ ] Gingivae: Upper
Lower
Retromolar trigone

Characteristics of Tumor

[ ] Exophytic

[ ] Superficial

[ ] Moderately infiltrating

[ ] Deeply infiltrating

[ ] Ulcerated

[ ] Extends to or overlies bone

[ ] Gross erosion of bone

[ ] Radiographic destruction of bone

Involvement of Neighboring Regions

[ ] Tonsillar pillar or soft palate

[ ] Nasal cavity or antrum

[ ] Nasopharynx

[ ] Pterygoid muscles

[ ] Soft tissues or skin of neck

Staged by _____ D.D.S./M.D.

FIG 9–1.
Clinical documentation of lesions of the lip and oral cavity.

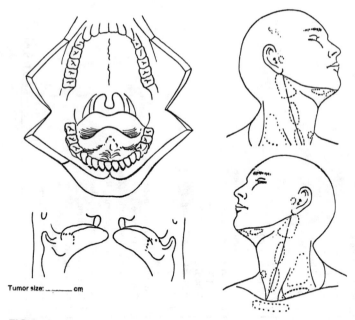

Tumor size: _____ cm

FIG 9–2.
Diagram for clinical documentation of primary tumor and involved lymph
nodes.

design of the definitive excision to follow. If the diagnosis of benign lesion is returned, this extensive procedure would not have been justified. On occasion, a very small (few millimeters) suspect lesion may be excised, inasmuch as wide local excision would compromise very few structures.

If the clinician has had minimal experience with malignant lesions, and a persistent clinical lesion is not highly suspect but the clinician is unsure of its nature, toluidine blue application may be used to help rule out a false negative clinical impression. Toluidine blue is a biologic stain that appears to stain malignant lesions preferentially over benign tumors or normal mucosa. Because toluidine blue may stain an inflammatory lesion, it is wise to wait 10 to 14 days after the discovery of an asymptomatic lesion, to allow benign inflammatory lesions to subside. Staining thereafter will produce few false positive results.

Toluidine blue may also be used to identify areas most likely to reveal the presence of malignancy on biopsy.

VIII. REFERRAL

A histologic diagnosis of severe dysplasia, carcinoma in situ, or invasive carcinoma requires that the lesion be treated. In general, asymptomatic, minimally developed lesions may be treated by wide local excision, which should not excessively compromise oral structures. However, on occasion, because of multicentricity or the presence of more than one primary cancer within a structure, as may occur in the soft palate, radiotherapy may be more advisable. In either case, small asymptomatic lesions are curable. If the clinician is not equipped by experience or background to treat the lesion, referral to the appropriate clinician is mandatory. A consultation request should be sent to a clinician with experience in treating oral and oropharyngeal cancer. In the consult, a statement should be made as to the location and appearance of the lesion, its size, biopsy results, and any other pertinent information related to the lesion.

BIBLIOGRAPHY

Eliezri YD: The toluidine blue test: An aid in the diagnosis and treatment of early squamous cell carcinomas of mucous membrane. *J Am Acad Dermatol* 1988; 28:1339–1349.

Mashberg A: Reevaluation of toluidine blue application as a diagnostic adjunct in the detection of asymptomatic oral squamous carcinoma. *Cancer* 1980; 46:758–763.

Mashberg A: Erythroplasia: The earliest of asymptomatic oral cancer. *J Am Dent Assoc* 1978; 96:615–620.

Mashberg A, Meyers H: Anatomic site and size of 222 asymptomatic oral squamous cell carcinomas: A continuing prospective study of oral cancer. II. *Cancer* 1976; 37:2149–2157.

Shedd DP: Clinical characteristics of early oral cancer. *JAMA* 1971; 215:955–956.

Chapter 10 _____

Squamous Cell Carcinoma

James J. Sciubba

_____

Squamous cell carcinoma accounts for approximately 4% of all cancers in men and 2% in women. This 2:1 ratio represents a significant shift from the earlier reported ratio of 3:1, probably due to the increased incidence of smoking by women. The overall incidence data convert to approximately 2% of all cancer-related deaths in men and 1% in women, with the total number of annual deaths due to oral cancer reaching nearly 9,500.

Squamous cell carcinoma of the oral cavity and oropharynx assumes many different appearances during its progression from a minimal or barely visible clinical lesion to a symptomatic lesion. By the time a carcinoma becomes symptomatic, producing pain or dysfunction, it usually is 1 to 2 cm in diameter, and frequently larger. It is not uncommon for a patient to be comparatively comfortable, with minimal dysfunction, until the lesion is 3 to 4 cm and has invaded deeper structures, such as muscles of the tongue, muscles of mastication, and/or the mandible.

Symptomatic lesions generally reveal some if not all of the following characteristics: induration, exophytic growth, ulceration, multiple surface changes including granularity, occasional

210

bleeding, keratin formation, inflammation, and interference with function. Invasion of bony structures may be seen on radiographs. At least 50% of patients have concomitant cervical lymphadenopathy, usually submandibular or jugulodigastric, due to metastasis.

These lesions and their sequelae can be considered late in the course of the cancer. It is now well established that cancer, from its initiation, may persist for a considerable time prior to becoming symptomatic. There is an apparent long asymptomatic phase during which the tumor enlarges. Therefore it behooves the clinician to develop a set of standards by which to diagnose early asymptomatic cancer, which displays none or few of the above signs and symptoms.

Staging is a useful method to relate outcome of treatment and survival to extent of disease at presentation, and may be used as a guide to prognosis. Clinical staging of oral carcinoma is based on the TNM system, where T refers to the size of the tumor in centimeters at its primary site of occurrence, N describes the presence of clinically palpable and potentially metastatic lymph nodes related to the primary tumor, and M describes the clinical and radiographic presence or absence of metastatic disease (Tables 10–1 and 10–2). A small diagram indicating the location of lesion is also helpful. If at all possible a

TABLE 10–1.

TNM System for Staging Oral
Squamous Cell Carcinoma

T: Tumor
T1: tumor <2 cm in diameter
T2: tumor 2 to 4 cm in diameter
T3: tumor >4 cm in diameter
T4: tumor invades adjacent
   structures
N: Node
N0: no palpable nodes
N1: ipsilateral palpable nodes
N2: contralateral or bilateral nodes
N3: fixed palpable nodes
M: Metastasis
M0: no distant metastasis
M1: Clinical or radiographic
   evidence of metastasis

TABLE 10–2.
TNM Staging System

Stage I	T1,N0,M0
Stage II	T2,N0,M0
Stage III	T3,N0,M0
	T1,N1,M0
	T2,N1,M0
	T3,N1,M0
Stage IV	T1,N2,M0
	T2,N2,M0
	T3,N2,M0
	T1,N3,M0
	T2,N3,M0
	T3,N3,M0
	T4,N0,M0
	Any M1

photograph of the lesion should be included for documentation purposes.

I. CARCINOMA OF LIPS

Carcinoma of the lips is far more common in the lower lip. In addition to pipe smoking as an important factor, the cause includes exposure to ultraviolet light. The growth rate of lower lip cancers tends to be slower than for upper lip cancers. The prognosis for lower lip lesions is generally good, whereas the prognosis for upper lip lesions of similar clinical stage is only fair.

Squamous cell carcinoma of the lip accounts for 25% to 30% of all oral cancers. Men are affected far more frequently than women, and the primary age at onset is 50 to 70 years. Most lesions tend to arise on the vermilion portion of the lip, with the clinical appearance often related to a chronic nonhealing ulcer or an exophytic and occasionally verrucous growth. Lesions of the lower lip tend to be well differentiated and slow growing, compared with less well differentiated, more rapidly growing lesions of the upper lip. Lower lip lesions tend to invade deeply late in the course of the disease, and correspondingly metastasis to submental and submandibular lymph nodes is uncommon for lower lip lesions in early clinical stages; this is not the case for upper lip lesions.

The prognosis for lower lip lesions less than 2 cm in diameter (T1) is excellent, with a cure rate for stage I and stage II lesions without regional lymph node metastasis greater than 90% with surgical or radiation therapy. Including all lesions of the lip, the 5-year determinant survival is approximately 80%, with a poorer prognosis in patients younger than 40 years.

II. CARCINOMA OF TONGUE

Carcinoma of the tongue is the most common intraoral malignancy, accounting for 25% to 40% of all oral carcinomas, excluding lip lesions. There is a predilection for men in the sixth through eighth decades.

After the asymptomatic early phase, deeper invasion of muscle and fascial spaces in later phases tends to produce pain or dysphagia and significant functional impairment. Clinically, lesions tend to be indurated and ulcerated. The middle third of the tongue is the most common site of origin of tongue cancer, with primary lesions at this site gaining access to the anterior tonsillar pillars, tonsillar fossa, and retromolar trigone, as well as the floor of the mouth. Lesions in the more posterior portions of the tongue may occasionally present with an exophytic growth pattern and overall bulky appearance. It is uncommon for primary lesions to involve the dorsum or the anterior free margin of the tongue, with the most prominent exception being carcinoma arising in syphilitic glossitis. Metastases from this site usually tend to involve the submandibular or jugulodigastric nodes initially; distant metastatic disease is relatively uncommon. The incidence of lymph node metastasis from carcinomas arising from the anterior third of the tongue occur less frequently than those arising in the middle third, whereas carcinomas involving the base of the tongue are associated with a high rate of metastasis to cervical lymph nodes on either side of the midline. Correspondingly, carcinomas involving the base of the tongue have a poorer prognosis than similar lesions involving the anterior two thirds of the tongue.

T1 or T2 lesions may be successfully treated with surgery and/or radiotherapy. The surgical approach for smaller lesions is intraoral; T3 and larger lesions often require mandibulotomy for access and adequacy of resection. Lesions approaching the gingiva or those that superficially extend into it usually require marginal mandibulectomy for a satisfactory en bloc removal. More massive lesions require composite resection, often with postoperative radiotherapy.

III. CARCINOMA OF FLOOR OF MOUTH

Carcinoma of the floor of the mouth is the second most common intraoral location for squamous cell carcinomas and accounts for up to 20% of such intraoral lesions. As with other forms of intraoral carcinoma, older men are predominantly affected, especially those with a history of heavy smoking and drinking habits. Clinical presentation is often that of an indurated, nonhealing, painless ulcer, which is usually preceded by erythroplakia with or without a keratotic component. The anterior segment of the floor of the mouth in the paramedian location is the most frequent site of origin. With progression the lesion adopts an exophytic or heavily granular to papillary appearance, and is usually advanced when first noted clinically. Deep infiltration is often present at the time of diagnosis. This infiltration can extend to the genioglossus muscle, the mandible, or into the root of the tongue. Floor of mouth lesions that are advanced at presentation are notoriously difficult to control, with metastases to cervical lymph nodes usually occurring late in the course of the disease, compared with similar size lesions of the tongue.

Superficial lesions of early clinical stage can often be successfully resected intraorally. Lesions of superficial pattern may be resected and closed primarily; deeper lesions approaching the gingiva may require a marginal mandibulectomy, with preservation of the outer cortex of the mandible. If the mandible is more extensively involved, segmental mandibulectomy should be performed. Use of skin or composite grafts as well as regional flaps or free microvascular flaps may be necessary for lesions of advanced clinical stage.

IV. CARCINOMA OF GINGIVA AND BUCCAL MUCOSA

Carcinoma of the gingiva and buccal mucosa accounts for less than 10% of all oral malignancies. Lesions involving the gingiva tend to arise in the premolar and molar regions, with the mandible the more frequent site. Clinical presentation usually is that of a nodular to plaquelike lesion, often with granular to exophytic surface features and a superficial spreading tendency. Most lesions tend to be well keratinized, and in approximately half the cases involve the underlying bone. The incidence of metastasis is approximately 30%.

Evaluation of exophytic lesions of the gingiva and buccal mucosa must include verrucous carcinoma. This is a separate type of squamous cell carcinoma, usually associated with the use of chewing tobacco. Presentation generally is that of a broad-based wartlike mass, often with a white tufted surface. The lesion tends to grow slowly, and rarely metastasizes.

Verrucous carcinoma is best treated with wide surgical excision. Formerly, use of radiotherapy as a primary treatment method was discouraged because of concern for inducing undifferentiated carcinoma within the more well-differentiated primary tumor. More recently, however, radiotherapy has proved effective when delivered properly and in selected clinical cases. The overall prognosis for verrucous carcinoma is good stage for stage when compared with the usual type of squamous cell carcinoma.

V. DIFFERENTIAL DIAGNOSIS

Typical oral squamous cell carcinomas must be differentiated from chronic nonhealing ulcers due to trauma. An undiagnosed chronic ulceration must be considered potentially infectious until a biopsy or culture proves otherwise. On clinical grounds, differentiation of tuberculosis, syphilis, and deep fungal infections from oral squamous cell carcinoma can be difficult, if not impossible. Chronic injuries such as factitial trauma can mimic squamous carcinoma. Lesions of the palate such as necrotizing sialometaplasia, midline granuloma, and Wegener's granulomatosis can often appear similar to squamous carcinoma.

VI. TREATMENT

Oral cancers are generally treated best with surgery and/or radiation therapy. Small lesions such as T1 and T2 (stage I and stage II) carcinomas are typically treated with surgery alone, with radiation therapy held in abeyance or as a backup if recurrence is observed. Similar rates of cure, however, are documented for T1 (stage I) lesions using surgical methods or radiotherapy. Overall, the factors that determine treatment usually relate to location, clinical stage, histologic type, and experience and skill of the therapy team. Larger lesions, such as stage III and stage IV, are usually treated with surgery followed by radiation. Elective or prophylactic neck dissection is often related to the philosophy of the primary surgeon, with stage II and larger lesions often treated with neck dissection.

The radiation dosage necessary to successfully treat squamous cell carcinoma either as a primary or adjunctive method ranges from 4,000 to 7,000 rads (cGy). Dosage is approximately 6,000 to 6,500 rads (cGy) delivered over 6 to 7 weeks. Tumorcidal doses of radiation carry signifcant side effects, both temporary and permanent. Temporary side effects include mucosal ulceration/mucositis, pain, dysgeusia/hypogeusia, candidiasis, dermatitis, alopecia, and cutaneous erythema. More permanent side effects include xerostomia with resultant radiation-type cervical caries, cutaneous telangiectasia, atrophy of the oral mucosa and the skin, permanent alopecia, and potential for osteoradionecrosis.

In general, the prognosis for oral squamous cell carcinoma depends on histologic subtype and clinical stage of the tumor. Of these two factors, clinical stage is more important. With the presence of metastasis to regional lymph nodes the 5-year survival rate, regardless of location, is essentially reduced by 50%. The overall 5-year survival rate for oral squamous carcinoma is approximately 45% to 50%. However, if the neoplasm is detected early and treated promptly, the overall cure rate may be as high as 60% to 70%, and for lesions of the lower lip may reach 90%.

The overall prognosis for oral cancer must consider also an increased level of risk for development of second primary tumors. Such lesions do not represent persistent or recurrent disease but separate lesions involving the upper aerodigestive tract or other organ systems. Field effect or field cancerization is the single most important factor relative to this phenomenon when the same anatomically contiguous area becomes involved by a second primary tumor. However, carcinogenic exposure within the upper aerodigestive tract clearly accounts for the majority of second primary tumors. Recent clinical trials of orally administered 13-*cis*-retinoic acid indicate significantly reduced rates of second primary cancers of the upper aerodigestive tract and lungs.

Management of short- and long-term effects of radiation therapy must be considered for all patients receiving therapeutic doses of external and/or interstitial radiation therapy for malignant disease. Management of mucositis and mucosal ulceration may include rinses with a mixture of saline solution and baking soda, which often provides temporary relief. Chlorhexidine (0.12%) has been used effectively in some studies in reducing the intraoral bacterial concentration and in helping to reduce local counts of *Candida albicans*. For candidiasis, topical antifungal agents generally are helpful, but must be considered carefully because most contain high concentrations of sugar. Sugar can be devastating in a xerostomic environment, because it is related to dental breakdown.

The long-term effects of radiation therapy beyond 18 to 24 months must be managed extremely carefully in that the attendant xerostomia and potential tooth breakdown can result in pulpal exposure and subsequent periapical disease. Periodontal disease with deep pocket formation likewise can produce similar problems as periapical disease can and must be managed diligently. Approximately 6 months after completion of radiotherapy demonstrable vascular compromise is evident, and by 2 years is completely manifest. Tooth extractions within the irradiated field, in particular within the mandible, pose a high risk for development of osteoradionecrosis. This tissue change remains permanent in that the radiation-induced intrabony vascular compromise leads to tissue hypoxia and a hypocellular and hypovascular state. The clinical manifestations are poor or absent healing and bony remodeling relative to tooth extractions or any form of bony surgical manipulation. Therefore prevention remains the primary therapy, along with topical applications of fluoride, remineralizing solutions, dietary management, scrupulous oral hygiene, and frequent dental visits to monitor any incipient dental and periodontal disease.

BIBLIOGRAPHY

Batsakis JG: Surgical margins in squamous cell carcinomas. *Ann Otol Rhinol Laryngol* 1988; 97:213–214.

Blot WJ, McLaughlin JK, Winn DM: Smoking and drinking in relation to oral and pharyngeal cancer. *Cancer Res* 1988; 48:3282–3287.

Centers for Disease Control: Deaths from oral cavity and pharyngeal cancer: United States, 1987. *MMWR*, 1990; 39:457–459.

McCoy TD, Wynder EL: Etiological and preventive implications in alcohol carcinogenesis. *Cancer Res* 1979; 39:2844–2850.

Shafer WG, Waldron CA: Eythroplakia of the oral cavity. *Cancer* 1975; 36:1021–1028.

Silverman S Jr: Early diagnosis of oral cancer. *Cancer* 1988; 62:1796–1799.

Sliverman S Jr: *Oral Cancer*. New York, American Cancer Society, 1985.

Silverman S Jr, Gorsky M, Lozada F: Oral leukoplakia and malignant transformation: A followup study of 257 patients. *Cancer* 1984; 53:563–568.

Vikram H, Strong EW, Shah JP, et al: Failure at the primary site following multimodality treatment in advanced head and neck cancer. *Head Neck Surg* 1984; 6:720–723.

Waldron CA, Shafer WG: Leukoplakia revisited: A clinical pathologic study of 3256 oral leukoplakias. *Cancer* 1975; 36:1386–1392.

Wright BA, Wright JM, Binnie WH: *Oral Cancer: Clinical and Pathological Considerations*. Boca Raton, Fla, CRC Press, 1988.

Drug-Induced Oral Mucosal Lesions

Harry Lumerman
Paul D. Freedman
Stanley M. Kerpel

_____

Systemic or topical medications may induce lesions of the oral mucosa. The clinical appearance of these lesions may be distinctive, or they may resemble other well-established oral mucosal diseases, such as lichen planus. In most instances, withdrawal of the medication will result in gradual disappearance of the lesions. At times, topical steroids and/or antibacterial and antifungal medications will be necessary.

The following criteria can be used to establish a diagnosis of drug-induced oral mucosal lesions:

1. **History of drug or chemical administration** followed by the occurrence of oral mucosal lesions.
2. **Mucosal lesions** noted are known to occur secondary to intake of the drug in question, as described in the product insert information or *Physician's Desk Reference*.
3. **Gradual resolution of oral lesions** after discontinuance of suspect medication.
4. **Recurrence of lesions** with readministration of the medication.

I. DRUG-INDUCED ORAL MUCOSAL LESIONS

Contact mucositis
Allergic contact mucositis
Erythema multiforme
Lichenoid mucositis
Discolorations of oral mucosa
Candida infections
Gingival hyperplasia

A. Contact mucositis

Drugs that come in contact with the oral mucosa can induce either primary irritant contact mucositis (PICM) or allergic contact mucositis (ACM).

1. **Primary irritant contact mucositis** (PICM): Also known as chemical burn, PICM results from the drug's direct cytotoxic effect on the oral mucosa. Depending on the concentration of the chemical and duration of contact, oral lesions may occur within minutes or several hours later. Clinically these lesions may assume one or more of the following patterns:
   a. Localized erythema.
   b. Superficial, white adherent pseudomembrane.
   c. Necrotic slough.
   d. Ulceration.

   The **microscopic changes** seen during the early stages of PICM may include atrophy or ulceration of the epithelium, as well as scattered numbers of necrotic keratinocytes. Eventually, marked hydropic degeneration (intracellular edema) develops, and may lead to intraepithelial vesicle formation. Occasionally the intraepithelial vesicles contain neutrophils (microabscess formation). Within the underlying stroma is a superficial perivascular infiltrate composed of an admixture of lymphocytes, histiocytes, and neutrophils.

Drugs and chemicals reported to cause PICM through direct mucosal irritation include **alcohol, aspirin, chromic acid, creosote, dental impression materials, eugenol, gentian violet, mouthwashes, nonsteroidal anti-inflammatory medications, phenol, silver nitrate, and trichloracetic acid.**

2. **Allergic contact mucositis (ACM):** ACM is an immunologically mediated lesion that results from a delayed hypersensitivity reaction. As the term implies, these delayed hypersensitivity reactions take 24 to 96 hours to manifest clinically. Prior exposure to a drug is necessary to sensitize the patient before a mucosal reaction to the drug can be elicited.

The clinical appearance of ACM may include localized areas of erythema, edematous papules, vesicles or bullae, and ulcerations.

The immunologic mechanisms leading to ACM are initiated by previous contact with the offending drug. The drug acts as a hapten that combines with the mucosal epithelial proteins to form a complete antigen. Langerhans cells within the epithelium present the processed antigen to T lymphocytes. The T lymphocytes are thereby sensitized to the drug. Subsequent exposure to the drug induces a delayed hypersensitivity response. In this response, T lymphocytes and the secreted lymphokines produce erythema, edematous papules, vesicle formation, and ulceration.

The microscopic appearance of ACM shows marked spongiosis (intercellular edema) of the epithelium. In some areas the edema leads to intraepithelial vesicle formation (reticular degeneration). A subepithelial infiltrate of lymphocytes admixed at times with eosinophils is present, and often extends into the overlying epithelium (exocytosis). Within the superficial connective tissue is a perivascular infiltrate composed of lymphocytes, histiocytes, and variable numbers of eosinophils.

Drugs and chemicals reported to cause allergic oral mucositis include **bis-GMA composites, ceramic metal alloys, chewing gums, chewing tobacco, coffee, denture adhesives, gold, hard candies, impression materials, lipsticks, lozenges, methylmethacrylate, mouthwashes, nickel alloys, periodontal packs (dressings), silver amalgam, toothpastes, topical analgesics, and volatile oils.**

C. **Erythema multiforme**

Erythema multiforme is an acute, immunologically mediated hypersensitivity reaction that can be related to drug intake in as many as 40% of reported cases. Herpes simplex and *Mycoplasma* infections have been noted as predisposing factors. In a large number of cases the cause remains unknown.

Localized areas or the entire oral mucosa may be involved, with erythema, vesicles, bullae, necrotic slough, or ulcerations. Hemorrhagic crusting of the lips is common. The disease pattern is usually bilaterally symmetric.

A pathognomonic sign of erythema multiforme of the skin is the presence of bullae surrounded by an erythematous halo, leading to the formation of the typical "target lesion." This lesion, which is often not present in oral erythema multiforme, occurs mostly on the palms of the hands or the soles of the feet.

Histologic examination of epithelial cells reveals necrotic keratinocytes and intraepithelial or subepithelial bullae formation. Keratinocyte death results from the action or interaction of natural killer cells, cytotoxic T cells, macrophages, complement-fixing antibodies, and effector cells for antibody-dependent cytotoxicity.

The most commonly used drugs that have been associated with the production of oral erythema multiforme include **aminopyrines, barbiturates, captopril, carbamazepine, chlorpropamide, clindamycin, digitalis, iodides, isoniazid, marijuana, meprobamate, mercury, oral contraceptives, penicillin, phenophthalein, phenothiazines, phenytoin, salicylates, sulfonamides, tetracycline, and thiouracil.**

D. **Lichenoid mucositis**

A small number of oral lichen planus–like (lichenoid) lesions can be related to drug intake. Both the drug-induced lichenoid lesions and classic lichen planus can present clinically as keratotic, reticular plaques with areas of erosion. Identification of a drug cause is important, because the drug-induced lesions usually resolve or become asymptomatic when the causative drug is withdrawn.

Histologically, drug-induced lesions show features similar to classic lichen planus, such as parakeratosis, sawtooth rete ridges, loss of basal cells, and a bandlike subepithelial inflammatory infiltrate. In lichenoid mucositis, the subepithelial infiltrate is composed of a mixture of plasma cells and lymphocytes, whereas in classic lichen planus the infiltrate consists almost exclusively of lymphocytes. Other findings include exocytosis of inflammatory cells, submucosal eosinophils, perivasculitis, and occasional submucosal lymphoid nodule formation.

Drugs most commonly reported to cause oral lichenoid mucositis include **allopurinol, arsenic, bismuth, captopril, chloroquine, chlorothiazide, chlorpropamide, dapsone, furosemide, gold salts injections, mepacrine, nonsteroidal anti-inflammatory medications, *p*-aminosalicylic acid, phenothiazine, phenytoin, propranolol, quinidine, tetracycline, thiazides, tolbutamide, triprolidine, and mercury.**

E. **Discoloration of Oral Mucosa**

Several types of mucosal discoloration have been described, including black "hairy" tongue, slate gray mucosa, and yellow to light brown mucosa.

Black "hairy" tongue results in most cases from alteration in the oral bacterial flora or bacterial metabolic by-products. This change can be induced by antibiotics, such as penicillin and tetracycline, and by agents such as sodium perborate, hydrogen peroxide, bismuth subsalicylate (Pepto-Bismol), chlorhexidine, and methyldopa.

Slate gray discoloration of the oral mucosa may result from intake of chloroquine, minocycline, and amiodarone. **Yellow to light brown discoloration** may be associated with oral contraceptives and the use of nicotine.

Petechiae and purplish black, hemorrhagic ecchymotic patches can be seen in drug-induced thrombocytopenia.

Common drugs that have been found to induce thrombocytopenia include **allopurinol, acetaminophen, carbamazepine, cephalosporins, cimetidine, digitalis, meprobamate, methyldopa, phenylbutazone, phenytoin, quinidine, sulfonamides, tetracyclines, and tolbutamide.**

F. *Candida* infections

Broad-spectrum antibiotics and other antibacterial agents can alter the oral bacterial flora, resulting in the excessive proliferation of the fungus *Candida albicans*. In addition, topical and systemic steroids, oxygenating rinses, psychotropic drugs, and other xerostomic medications can predispose to oral candidiasis. The clinical lesions manifest as pseudomembranous ("milk curd"–like) plaques or diffuse erythematous macular patches.

G. **Gingival hyperplasia**

Three commonly used drugs, phenytoin, cyclosporine, and nifedipine, can induce a lobulated hyperplasia of the attached gingiva.

1. **Phenytoin-induced gingival hyperplasia**

Thirty percent to 70% of patients taking the anticonvulsant phenytoin exhibit gingival hyperplasia. The most common site of involvement is the anterior gingiva. Young patients are most often affected, and phenytoin-related gingival hyperplasia is seen rarely in patients older than 40 years.

It has been shown that phenytoin induces increased fibroblastic activity. The mechanism for such increased activity is not clear, but the presence of bacterial plaque is an important etiologic cofactor. In addition, subclasses of fibroblasts with high and low synthetic activity, which vary among individuals, play a role in the cause of this condition.

2. **Cyclosporine-induced gingival hyperplasia**
   Cyclosporine is a T cell immunosuppressant drug used to prevent graft rejection in organ transplant patients and also in the treatment of diabetes mellitus type I, rheumatoid arthritis, and psoriasis. According to the manufacturer of this drug, in clinical trials 16% of liver transplant patients, 9% of kidney transplant patients, and 5% of heart transplant patients demonstrated cyclosporine-associated gingival hyperplasia.

3. **Nifedipine-induced gingival hyperplasia**
   Nifedipine is a calcium channel blocking agent, with primary effect on vascular smooth muscle, producing coronary vasodilation and inhibition of coronary artery spasm. It is widely prescribed for all forms of angina pectoris and ventricular arrhythmias. Several cases of nifedipine-induced gingival hyperplasia have been reported. The mechanism of gingival overgrowth is unknown.

   Other calcium channel blocking agents also may produce gingival hyperplasia. Drugs reported less frequently to cause gingival hyperplasia are **diltiazem, primidone, phenobarbital, and valproate, and oral contraceptives.**

H. **Summary**

Numerous commonly prescribed drugs and locally applied chemicals can induce oral lesions. Some of these lesions may appear clinically similar to lichen planus (lichenoid mucositis). Other drug-induced oral conditions include contact mucositis, erythema multiforme, candidiasis, mucosal discoloration, and gingival hyperplasia.

The diagnosis is suggested by the patient's drug intake history. If a drug- or chemical-induced oral lesion is suspected, the initial investigation should be consultation with standard references, including the *Physician's Desk Reference* or product insert information. The observed oral lesion may have already been described as a side effect of the drug in question.

II. THERAPY

In many cases, adequate treatment may consist simply of withdrawal of the offending agent after consultation with the prescriber. In some instances, it may be possible to substitute another drug.

A. Contact mucositis

Therapy consists of withdrawal of the drug followed by symptomatic care, including saline/bicarbonate rinses. Topical steroid application may also be necessary to accelerate the healing process.

B. Erythema multiforme/lichenoid mucosal lesions

Therapy consists of withdrawal of the drug and use of topical or systemic steroids. Steroid treatment is indicated in cases of rapidly evolving lesions or widespread mucosal and cutaneous lesions at presentation.

C. Candidiasis

Therapy consists of withdrawal of the suspected drug and use of topical antifungal medication.

D. Gingival hyperplasia

Therapy consists of withdrawal of the drug and replacement with alternative compound if possible. Establishment of good oral hygiene is essential. Subsequent to drug withdrawal or change the hyperplastic tissue will remain if not surgically removed.

BIBLIOGRAPHY

Baker KA, Ettinger RC: Intraoral effects of drugs in elderly persons. *Geriodontics* 1985;1:111–116.

Bork K: *Cutaneous Side Effects of Drugs*. Philadelphia, WB Saunders, 1988.

Duxbury AJ: Systemic pharmacotherapy, in Jones JH, Mason DK (ed): *Oral Manifestations of Systemic Disease*. London, Bailliere Tindall, 1990, pp 411—479.

Gebel K, Hornstein OP: Drug induced oral erythema multiforme: Results of a long term retrospective study. *Dermatologica* 1984;168:35–40.

Hay KD, Reade PC: Spectrum of oral disease induced by drugs and other bioactive agents. *Drugs* 1983;26:268–277.

Konstantinidis AB, Markopoulos A, Trigonides G: Ampicillin induced erythema multiforme *J Oral Med* 1985;40:168–170.

Lederman D, Lumerman H, Reuben S, et al: Gingival hyperplasia associated with nifedipine therapy. *Oral Surg Oral Med Oral Pathol* 1984;57:620–622.

Lever WF, Schaumberg-Lever G: Histopathology of the skin, ed 5. Philadelphia, JB Lippincott, 1975, pp 92–100, 159–268.

Lozada-Nur F, Huang MZ, Zhou G: Open preliminary clinical trials of clobetasol proprionate ointment in adhesive paste for treatment of chronic oral vesiculoerosive diseases. *Oral Surg Oral Med Oral Pathol* 1991; 71:283–287.

Lozada-Nur F, Silverman S Jr: Topically applied fluocinonide in adhesive base in the treatment of oral vesiculoerosive diseases. *Arch Dermatol* 1981; 116:898–901.

Mobacken H, Hersle K, Sloberg K, et al: Oral lichen planus: Hypersensitivity to dental restoration material. *Contact Dermatitis* 1984;10:11–15.

Schechtman RL, Archard HO, Cox D: Oropharyngeal candidiasis associated with steroid-containing inhalers. *NY State Dent J* 1986;24–26.

Shafer WG, Hine MK, Levy BM: *A Textbook of Oral Pathology,* ed 4. Philadelphia, WB Saunders, 1983, pp 582–588.

Tyldesley WR, Rotter E: Gingival hyperplasia induced by cyclosporin-A. *Br Dent J* 1984;157:305–309.

Wright JM: Oral manifestations of drug reactions. *Dent Clin North Am* 1984;28:529–543.

Chapter 12 _____

Control of Anxiety and Apprehension

Robert M. Peskin

_____

I. SELECTION OF APPROPRIATE ANESTHESIA
A. Knowledge of the patient
Knowing the patient under treatment is essential to selection of appropriate anesthesia. Factors important in

formulating this evaluation include (1) the patient's age, (2) complete review of current illness, (3) past medical history, and (4) assessment of physical status. Such review will produce a classification of risk as defined by the American Society of Anesthesiologists (ASA).

1. **Age** plays a very important role. Among other factors, it can identify a patient's ability to cooperate, as well as the inability to reasonably predict a response to medication. Age may preclude the establishment of an intravenous route for the administration of drugs, necessitating an alternate route (e.g., oral, rectal, submucosal, intramuscular, inhalation).

2. **Complete review of current illness** is basic to the formulation of realistic and appropriate anesthetic and sedation therapies. The evaluation includes the following considerations:

   a. **Chief complaint** (CC) is essential in determining the anesthetic method to be used.

      (1) **Dental presentation** is considered in terms of:

         a. Level of urgency. Intense, refractory pain requires less management preparation if anesthesia is to be used. In instances where consciousness is altered and the airway is not secured (e.g., by an endotracheal tube) a minimal requirement is an empty stomach, even when past medical history would not otherwise have an impact on the choice of anesthetic method.

         b. Presence of severe local infection can significantly compromise the airway and create additional anesthetic considerations.

      (2) **Level of anxiety and apprehension** will influence choice of anesthetic method.

   b. **Past medical history** (PMH) may have a significant impact on anesthetic management. Such review goes beyond the simple check-off form completed and signed by the patient. An oral dialog between the dentist (not an auxiliary) and the patient (or parent or legal guardian) will clarify and provide additional detail on positive information elicited by the check-off form (if used). Direct questioning is required for:

(1) **Review of past surgical/anesthetic history,** including anesthetic complications experienced by the patient or any blood relative.

(2) **Review of systems** (ROS), including but not limited to respiratory, gastrointestinal, genitourinary, cardiovascular, neurologic, musculoskeletal, and endocrine systems.

(3) **Allergy history,** including substances the patient is allergic to and the nature of the allergic phenomenon.

(4) **Detailed drug history,** including prescription and over-the-counter drugs and recreational drugs taken, how long (months, years), dosage, frequency, etc.

(5) **Smoking history,** including frequency and duration of current or former habit.

(6) **Alcohol consumption,** including frequency and quantity. The patient who relates only social consumption of alcohol may be socializing on a daily basis.

(7) **Review of past dental experiences** that may contribute to a patient's apprehension or anxiety. A full understanding of factors that have affected the patient's perception of dentistry from an historical perspective will prove invaluable when formulating an anesthetic approach.

c. **Physical examination** of the patient completes the assessment of ASA risk, and includes evaluation of blood pressure, pulse rate, heart, lungs, and height and weight.

Emerging from the entire review will be a classification of risk, according to the ASA Physical Status Classification System, updated in 1962 (Table 12–1).

Examples of disease classified as ASA II in-

TABLE 12– 1.

ASA Physical Status Classification Systems*

ASA I: No systemic disease (normal healthy patient).

ASA II: Mild to moderate systemic disease.

ASA III: Severe systemic disease that limits activity but is not incapacitating.

ASA IV: Severe systemic disease that limits activity and is a constant threat to life.

ASA V: Moribundity (patient not expected to survive 24 hours with or without operation).

ASA E: Emergency operation (used to modify one of the above classifications, e.g., ASA E-III).

*Data from American Society of Anesthesiologists: *Anesthesiology* 1963; 24:111.

clude controlled hypertension, well-controlled insulin-dependent diabetes, hepatitis B in a patient who is antigen positive, and heavy smoking accompanied by chronic bronchitis. In patients with multiple compromises, such as hypertension plus diabetes, a greater risk category should be assigned.

It is the informed clinician's responsibility to weigh the results of evaluation of the ASA I or II patient and determine if additional preoperative testing is indicated. Certain laboratory or function tests may be appropriate. A consulting physician may be necessary. In ASA III risk or higher, it is prudent and essential for the practitioner to pursue consultation with a medical colleague prior to administering therapy.

B. **Management requirements**

In establishing management requirements, determination of the level of patient apprehension and anxiety is necessary. Equally important is assessment of existing handicap(s), either emotional or physical, and the presence of a developmental disability.

1. **Anxiety level** can be quantified by one of three self-report measures: Dental Anxiety Scale (DAS), State-Trait Anxiety Inventory (STAI), Visual Analogue Scale (VAS).

The DAS and STAI have been extensively researched and have proved helpful in assessing anxiety. The VAS, although less extensively researched, correlates well with these scales and indices and is more readily incorporated into an initial intake form completed by the patient (Fig 12–1). Regardless of the actual test utilized, some assessment of anxiety preoperatively will offer appropriate insight into the impact that anxiety will have on patient management.

2. **Assess the mentally retarded patient's** ability to feed, dress, and toilet. Where cooperation of the patient is essential, inability may preclude the use of a given anesthetic method. Diminished or complete lack of ability in any of these areas will offer insight.

C. **The nature of anticipated treatment**
   1. **If an involved technical procedure is contemplated,** where patient movement will undermine the predictability of results, a technique limiting patient movement is considered.
   2. **The projected duration of a given procedure** is an equally important consideration. Procedures lasting more than 3 hours may require use of general anesthetic with a protected airway provided by endotracheal intubation.

   Once these considerations are evaluated, the nature of the anesthetic modality can be identified. Attention can then be directed to the practitioner who will provide the anesthetic and the site of administration.

VISUAL ANALOGUE SCALE

Please mark your current level of anxiety or nervousness with a cross (X) on the dotted line

I I
(100 mm)

Totally calm   Worst Fear
and relaxed   imaginable

FIG 12–1.
Visual Analogue Scale.

D. Practitioner training

The safety and efficacy of anesthesia and sedation performed by trained dentists depend predominantly on the drugs, doses, and routes of administration. These three variables determine the level of patient consciousness, degree of monitoring needed, and potential morbidity and mortality associated with the anesthetic procedure.

Dentists may administer oral premedication, largely on the basis of predoctoral training in pharmacology. The use of inhalation sedation with nitrous oxide plus oxygen is another example. An increasing number of states limit use of any anesthetic method to those individuals who satisfy postdoctoral educational criteria. The intravenous method appropriately is limited to individuals with formal advanced training, and in most states requires a separate permit or certificate.

E. Treatment setting

Treatment may be carried out in (1) the practitioner's office, (2) an ambulatory care facility, or (3) an inpatient hospital. This decision is based on clinical judgment and experience. For example, a patient with a history of frequent episodes of asthma may be best managed in a hospital or ambulatory surgical setting, whereas an individual who has a vague history of asthma, with no attacks in the last 5 years, may be adequately managed in the practitioner's office. The final determination is based on (1) the patient, (2) the anesthetist, and (3) the office setting, as well as the limitations of these factors. The anesthetist must have the ability to manage unanticipated untoward sequelae.

II. OVERVIEW OF AMBULATORY ANESTHESIA

Single drugs in differing doses or differing combinations of drugs can result in different states of altered consciousness. One patient's response to a given drug regimen is not always predictably the same as another patient's, nor is the response the same in any patient under differing circumstances.

A recent study found that 82 different drugs and drug combinations are used by dental practitioners with advanced training in general anesthesia and deep sedation.

A. **Oral premedication**

Several preparations that can be used as premedication in adults, either prior to parenteral sedation or alone prior to an operative procedure. Available oral premedication most often used in adults is **diazepam,** a benzodiazepine. Other medications include barbiturates, nonbenzodiazepine-nonbarbiturates, and hypnotics, such as the orally administered agents, which include **chloral hydrate, hydroxyzine, promethazine, lorazepam, meperidine, diphenhydramine, pentobarbital, and ethinamate.**

B. **Nitrous oxide**

Nitrous oxide used in conjunction with oxygen provides an inhalation sedative agent that has a remarkable safety record. A minimal concentration of 30% oxygen is mandatory with the use of nitrous oxide.

C. **Parenterally administered drugs**

Parenteral drugs are classified as:

1. Benzodiazepines.
2. Narcotics.
3. Other anxiolytic agents (e.g., phenothiazines, butyrophenones).
4. Dissociative anesthetics.
5. Antisialogogues/anticholinergics.
6. Barbiturates.

Some of these agents can be administered intramuscularly. The most frequently selected agents for the IM route are **midazolam** and **ketamine,** and less often a narcotic, such as **meperidine.**

The most reliable and predictable route of administration is **intravenous infusion.** Often intravenous agents are supplemented by nitrous oxide and oxygen. If necessary, oral premedication may be given to alter the mood of the patient prior to the establishment of an intravenous infusion.

D. It is important that in the absence of general anesthesia, local anesthesia (most frequently of the amide classification) is absolutely essential to the success of any sedative technique.

III. COMMON ANESTHETIC AGENTS

Anesthesia is defined as the loss of sensation in a part or in the body generally, induced by the administration of a drug. Therefore, if surgical stimulation does not elicit a response where local anesthesia has not been administered, a state of general anesthesia must exist. Similarly, if sedation is to be effective and successful, sound local anesthetic techniques must be used. This demands a thorough familiarity with the properties of the various anesthetic agents currently available, including onset of action, duration of action, and potency.

A. Benzodiazepines

The most common premedication agent is the benzodiazepine **diazepam** (Valium). A recent study indicated its use an an oral premedicant to be 2.5 times greater than any other oral premedicant. A specific advantage of oral diazepam is its relatively rapid absorption, within 1 to 2 hours. Mean elimination half-life for the agent is 27 to 37 hours. Diazepam is considered an excellent antianxiety, sedative, and hypnotic agent, and is often the drug of choice because of its efficacy and safety.

Other oral premedicants include **chloral hydrate, hydroxyzine, promethazine, lorazepam, meperidine, diphenhydramine, and pentobarbital.** Either alone or in conjunction with benzodiazepines, hypnotics such as ethinamate (Valmid) can be effective. Although this agent is not effective for sleep disorders after repeated dosages beyond 7 days, as a premedication it has some interesting properties. Its onset of action is quite rapid, with effects visible within 20 minutes. Elimination half-life is 2½ hours.

The combination of **diazepam plus ethinamate** is effective premedication for the extremely anxious patient, in whom it may be impossible to establish an intravenous route. Given **in the office** 30 minutes prior to the start of a procedure, it will provide excellent sedation and reduce the quantity of intravenous agent(s) necessary. Caution must be exercised, because these agents, either alone or in combination, can result in a state of deep sedation or even general anesthesia.

For intravenous use, benzodiazepines are the agents of choice because of their antianxiety, sedative, and hypnotic qualities. They produce excellent amnesia and muscle relaxant effects. They are considered to have distinct advantages over nonbenzodiazepines when considering adverse reactions, development of tolerance, drug dependence, drug interactions, and lethality associated with overdose. The benzodiazepines are by far the most commonly used intravenous sedative agents in use.

The most commonly used intravenous benzodiazepine is diazepam. The well-documented relatively high incidence of thrombophlebitis and venous thrombosis associated with intravenous diazepam is its chief disadvantage. Recently, midazolam has been introduced. The literature lists several advantages over diazepam, including faster onset of action, fast recovery, enhanced amnesic qualities, and reduced incidence of thrombophlebitis and venous thrombosis.

The introduction of midazolam should be viewed with caution. When first marketed it was thought to have twice the potency of diazepam; however, recent warnings from the manufacturer advise of a potency of three to four times that of diazepam. In untrained hands, use of the drug in a similar manner as diazepam can cause untoward complications, including respiratory depression and subsequent cardiovascular collapse.

B. **Narcotics**

Beyond the use of benzodiazepines, many who use sedative techniques rely on intravenous narcotics, primarily the opioid agonists. The agents most frequently used are **meperidine, morphine, and fentanyl.** The intravenous agents increase the pain threshold while exhibiting analgesic qualities. They are also sedatives, and create a state of euphoria. The advantage of narcotics over other agents is their reversibility. They are currently the only drug group known to be 100% reversible when the antagonist, **naloxone,** is administered.

Narcotics are not without disadvantage. Respiratory depression can occur as a direct effect on the central nervous system. Narcotics can cause a higher incidence of nausea and vomiting. Fentanyl has been reported to cause stiff chest syndrome. Meperidine is known to be responsible for histamine release. In addition, newer synthetic agonist-antagonist narcotics, including **butorphanol** (Stadol) and **nalbuphine** (Nubain) are also available. As a result of their antagonistic qualities, the use of these agents could be devastating to patients with a history of illicit drug use.

C. **Phenothiazines**

Other psychosedative agents, when added to an intravenous drug regimen, permit establishment of an appropriate sedative baseline. One category of agents is the phenothiazines. **Promethazine** and **promazine** are two such agents that potentiate the effect of other sedative agents. In addition to their psychosedative qualities, they possess antiemetic properties. Caution should be exercised against hypotension.

D. **Butyrophenones**

Another group of agents that enhance the overall sedative effect include the butyrophenones, such as **droperidol.** In fact, use of droperidol in combination with the narcotic fentanyl is the basis of neuroleptanesthesia and neuroleptanalgesia.

Problems with the use of droperidol include prolonged onset and duration of action. Many patients have reported restlessness and agitation. Some have observed an inability to verbalize and increase of inward anxiety resulting from the use of the agent.

E. **Anticholinergics/antisialogogues**

Anticholinergics/antisialogogues have been used as part of an intravenous technique. **Atropine** and **glycopyrrolate** are used primarily for control of secretions. In addition, they are vagolytic in that they counter the bradycardic effects of other anesthetic agents. Atropine, with rapid onset of action, will cause reflex tachycardia. Glycopyrrolate has a more subtle onset of action and blocks the bradycardic effects without causing significant reflex tachycardia.

In addition to these qualities, **Scopolamine** crosses

the blood-brain barrier and increases the depth of sedation. Because it may cause dissociation and hallucinations, use of the agent is discouraged in patients younger than 6 years or older than 65 years, even though these effects are somewhat reversible with physostigmine.

F. **Dissociative anesthetics**

Among the dissociative anesthetic group, **ketamine** has several applications. It is considered an induction agent for anesthesia, and can be used intramuscularly as a sedative agent as well. It is ideal for use in the recalcitrant patient who will not allow an intravenous infusion to be established. In lower dosages intravenously, it can be useful as an adjunct to a sedation technique. Ketamine may cause hallucinations. In addition, a marked increase in secretions occurs. The absence of respiratory depression and apparent minimal impact on blood pressure makes it a very useful adjunct.

G. **Barbiturates**

No discussion of intravenous sedation is complete without discussion of the barbiturates. As a group, these agents possess a broad duration of action. The ultrashort-acting agents, such as **methohexital, thiopental sodium and thiamylal,** circulate and are eliminated rapidly. The short-acting barbiturates have a longer duration of action.

The ultrashort nature of methohexital makes it the ultimate component of many techniques. It can obliterate response to painful stimuli by inducing general anesthesia for short periods. However, barbiturates in general are not effective in increasing pain threshold. In fact, given alone, they may act to actually decrease pain threshold, thus increasing the perception of pain.

Disadvantages include the absence of available reversal agents and the cumulative effect in obese patients. When used as a sole agent in intermittent boluses, patients tend to drift in and out of deep states of sedation/anesthesia. For this reason, establishment of a sedative baseline with other agents supplemented by intermittent use of barbiturates for short periods, where increased painful stimuli are anticipated, (e.g., local anesthesia administration, tooth elevation) is a more appropriate indication for its use.

IV. PHARMACOLOGIC DESENSITIZATION

To complete the discussion of the overall management of the anxious and apprehensive patient, consider treatment approaches that will over time allow for the continued management of an individual patient. Getting the anxious individual into the dental office for the first time is often an accomplishment. For that patient to return voluntarily for continued treatment at a later time may be impossible.

An approach to accomplish this goal incorporates both psychologic and pharmacologic methods. This particular strategy relies on the development of a trusting relationship between the patient and the clinician. It allows for the patient to be given control of the dental situation while recognizing that certain stimuli may be stressful and require available coping mechanisms. It incorporates positive reinforcement and gives fearful patients a realistic approach for continued dental therapy.

Although only recently coined, **pharmacologic desensitization** is a concept that has been observed. It has been recognized where decreasing depths of sedation during subsequent appointments have been required, while allowing the patient control of presenting aversive stimuli and thereby providing repeated positive experiences.

With pharmacologic desensitization, patients are relaxed with sedative agents. This is not unlike systematic desensitization whereby individuals are relaxed with various relaxation techniques. The drug regimen used is based on patient response. If during a given appointment a patient expresses heightened anxiety, additional medication can be administered.

This approach is based on the progressive unmasking of aversive stimuli. Initially, all stimuli are masked by the use of pharmacologic agents. At subsequent visits decreasing depths of sedation are provided, giving the patient an increased awareness of the reality of the dental treatment setting. As treatment progresses, patients learn to cope with an increased awareness of the procedures by stepwise elimination of the sedative regimen.

This phenomenon, which accompanies parenteral sedation techniques, is useful in fearful patients, permitting them to overcome anxiety. It is a behavioral strategy that over multiple visits will improve the efficacy of treatment and decrease the time necessary to overcome the patient's fear of dentistry.

BIBLIOGRAPHY

American Dental Association, Department of State Government Affairs: *States that Regulate Administration of Anesthesia, Conscious Sedation and Nitrous Oxide*. Chicago, The Association, 1989.

American Medical Association, Division of Drugs: *AMA Drug Evaluations,* ed 5. Chicago, The Association, 1983.

American Society of Anesthesiologists: New classification of physical status. *Anesthesiology* 1963;24:111.

American Society of Oral Surgeons, Committee on Anesthesia: ASOS anesthesia morbidity and mortality survey. *JOS* 1974;32:733– 738.

Ash HL: Anesthesia's dental heritage. *Anesth Prog* 1985;32:25–29.

Bennett CR, in *Monheim's Local Anesthesia and Pain Control in Dental Practice,* ed 7. St Louis, CV Mosby, 1984.

Bergman SA: The benzodiazepine receptor. *Anesth Prog* 1986;33:213– 219.

Corah NL, O'Shea RM: Patient and dentist selection in general practice, in Moretti R, Ayer WA (eds): *The President's Conference on the Dentist-Patient Relationship and the Management of Fear, Anxiety and Pain*. Chicago, American Dental Association, 1983, pp 3–9.

Department of Health and Human Services: Warning reemphasized in midazolam labeling. *FDA Drug Bull* 1987;17:5.

Department of Health and Human Services: Boxed warning added to midazolam labeling. *FDA Drug Bull* 1988;18:15–16.

Dionne RA, Gift HC: Drugs used for parenteral sedation in dental practice. *Anesth Prog* 1988;35:199–205.

Dionne RA: Pharmacologic consideration in the training of dentists in anesthesia and sedation. *J Dent Educ* 1989;53:297–299.

Johnson JV: Prevention of venous complications from intravenous anesthesia. *Anesth Prog* 1987;34:3–5.

Kurz-Kummerle S, Melamed BG, Kaplan LR, et al: Dental students' anxiety as it influences child patients' fear behaviors, in Moretti R, Ayer WA (eds): *The President's Conference on the Dentist-Patient Relationship and the Management of Fear, Anxiety and Pain.* Chicago, American Dental Association, 1983, pp 16–21.

Luyk NH, Beck FM, Weaver JM: A visual analogue scale in the assessment of dental anxiety. *Anesth Prog* 1988;35:121–123.

Luyk NH, Boyle MA, Ward-Booth RP: Evaluation of the anxiolytic and amnestic effects of diazepam and midazolam for minor oral surgery. *Anesth Prog* 1987;34:37–42.

McCarthy FM: *Emergencies in Dental Practice: Prevention and Treatment,* ed 3. Philadelphia, WB Saunders, 1979.

Malamed SF: *Sedation: A Guide to Patient Management,* ed 2. St Louis, CV Mosby, 1989.

Moore PA, Peskin RM, Pierce C: Pharmacologic desensitization for dental phobias: Clinical observations. *Anesth Prog* 1990;37:308–311.

National Institutes of Health: Consensus development conference statement on anesthesia and sedation in the dental office. *J Am Dent Assoc* 1985;11:90–93.

Weinstein P: The study of interactions with child patients, in Moretti R, Ayer WA (eds): *The President's Conference on the Dentist-Patient Relationship and the Management of Fear, Anxiety and Pain.* Chicago, American Dental Association, 1983, pp 10–15.

Chapter 13 _____

Drug Interactions

Frederick A. Curro

_____

Drugs most widely prescribed by dentists are used to treat infection or pain. In rank order from the 1988 Annual Prescription Survey, these drugs include **antibiotics** (penicillin V potassium [V-Cillin-K], tetracycline, erythromycin, potassium phenoxymethyl penicillin [Pen-Vee-K], **narcotic analgesics** (acetaminophen with codeine), **nonsteroidal anti-inflammatory drugs** (ibuprofen), **nonnarcotic analgesics** (acetaminophen), and **fluorides** (Phos-Flur). Prescribing a drug to elicit an effect at a peripheral effector end organ such as the tooth embraces all of the complex physiologic and pharmacologic principles affecting a biological system and must be viewed as such, that is, systemically.

I. DRUG INTERACTIONS

Drugs exist systemically in equilibrium as bound and free. It is the free concentration that is related to the drugs' active pharmacologic effect. The free concentration of drug or its active drug metabolite may be altered as a result of: (1) direct chemical or physical interactions, (2) altered gastrointestinal absorption, (3) binding to plasma or tissue proteins, (4) binding to receptor sites, (5) induction or inhibition of drug-metabolizing enzymes, (6) acid-base imbalance affecting drug distribution and clearance, and (7) drug interaction affecting renal clearance and other modes of excretion.

Patients who are medically compromised by any disease affecting primarily or secondarily the organs of absorption, metabolism, or excretion should be considered at risk for adverse drug interaction. Patients requiring multiple drug therapy are at an even greater risk. Both extremes of age, pediatric and geriatric, can affect drug action in the medically compromised patient. Bioequivalence and the pharmacokinetics of the medications prescribed can be a predisposing pharmaceutical factor and should be considered, especially in the medically compromised patient.

The role of protein binding in altered states has the greatest potential to elicit a drug interaction. The three major proteins responsible for drug binding in plasma are albumin, α_1-acid glycoprotein (AAG), and the lipoproteins. Drugs may bind to more than one plasma protein. Albumin is the major binding protein, and constitutes about 60% of the total plasma protein concentration. Most acidic drugs are bound in plasma to albumin, and recent work has shown that the principal binding protein for a large number of basic or cationic drugs is AAG. The medical conditions identified below are those in which patients would seek ambulatory dental care. Decreased albumin exists in renal disease, heptic disease, inflammatory disease, malnutrition, and malignancy; in the elderly and in pregnant women. Increased AAG levels are seen in infection, Crohn's disease, renal transplantation, chronic pain, malignancy, rheumatoid arthritis, ulcerative colitis. Oral contraceptives and pregnancy can decrease AAG levels.

II. GERIATRIC CONSIDERATIONS

The causes of adverse drug reactions in the elderly are primarily due to:

1. Inadequate clinical assessment.
2. Excessive prescribing:
   a. Patient pressure.
   b. Pharmaceutical company pressure.
   c. Therapeutic enthusiasm.
   d. Overenergetic treatment.
   e. Inappropriate treatment.
3. Inadequate supervision of long-term medication.
4. Altered pharmacokinetics and pharmacodynamics
5. Lack of compliance

Drug absorption has not been a systematic problem in the elderly despite evidence that increased gastric pH, reduction in absorbing cells, decreased splanchnic blood flow, and decreased gastrointestinal motility occur in many older individuals. In contrast, postabsorptive distribution does tend to differ in older patients. The direction of change, however, is not predictable on the basis of a drug's physico-chemical characteristics alone. In general, the distribution volume for fat-soluble drugs increases in the aged, and the opposite is true for water-soluble drugs. Similarly, serum albumin levels decline and AAG levels increase in the very old, increasing or decreasing in the free concentrations of acidic and basic drugs, respectively. The degree of change depends on the extent of drug binding to these proteins and other disposition mechanisms. The application of these trends to individual cases, however, must be adjusted for other factors, such as heart failure, edema, renal failure, dehydration, and drug interactions.

The effects of age on the metabolic disposition of drugs by the liver are unpredictable. To be sure, liver mass and blood flow to the liver decline with age. Thus the first-pass removal of drugs with high hepatic extraction ratios, such as lidocaine and propranolol, may be reduced. In addition, there is some evidence that liver microsomal oxidative activity is impaired in the elderly, but no significant alterations in conjugation reactions have been observed. It should be noted, however, that the evidence varies a great deal and that genetic and environmental factors often contribute more to differences in drug metabolism than does age.

The most consistent physiologic change associated with aging is a decline in renal function. This involves renal blood flow, glomerular filtration rate, and tubular secretion. As a result, drugs that are excreted substantially by the kidney regularly exhibit decreased plasma clearance in the elderly. This is particularly important for drugs with narrow therapeutic ratios, such as digoxin, quinidine, procainamide, aminoglycosides, and chlorpropamide. It is also important to note that renal function cannot be estimated in elderly patients by serum creatinine values alone, because production of this metabolite is reduced in this population by virtue of smaller muscle mass. For clinical purposes, however, formulas and nomograms that include an age term are available for this purpose. The ability to concentrate urine and conserve sodium also declines with age, which may have an important effect on homeostatic responses to drug-induced perturbations.

The characteristics of the geriatric consideration relative to drug disposition and responses include:

1. **Reduced renal function:** Accumulation of renally cleared drugs.
2. **Reduced serum albumin and increased AAG glycoprotein levels:** Changes in percent free drug, volume of distribution, and measured levels of bound drugs.
3. **Relative increase in body fat:** Increased distribution volume of fat-soluble drugs.
4. **Reduction in lean body mass and total body water:** Decreased distribution volume of water-soluble drugs.

5. **Reduction in liver metabolizing capacity:** Accumulation of metabolized drugs.
6. **Increased sensitivity to CNS drugs:** Adverse effects.
7. **Decreased cardiac reserve:** Potential for heart failure.
8. **Decreased baroreceptor sensitivity:** Tendency to orthostatic hypotension.
9. **Decreased vital capacity and maximum breathing capacity:** Increased risk from blockade and CNS depression.
10. **Oversecretion of antidiuretic hormone:** Potential for water intoxication.
11. **Concurrent illness:** Disease interactions.
12. **Multiple drugs:** Drug interactions.
13. **Large interindividual variations:** Wide dose range.

III. **GENERIC DRUGS**

The use of generic drugs, especially the older pharmaceutical drugs that are relatively simple to manufacture, have a demonstrated historical track record for clinical efficacy. Approval of generic drugs is primarily based on comparative in vivo bioavailability or bioequivalence studies. The production of generic drugs follows the development of innovative drugs by the pharmaceutical industry. The government's current bioequivalence education criteria allow generic drugs to be approved when the mean values are within ±20% of a reference product. This bioequivalence range should be considered when treating severe infections, for example, when the clinician would want to be assured of the pharmacologic characteristics of the reference product to achieve the necessary blood levels for onset of action and efficacy.

IV. **DRUG DISPOSITION IN OBESE PATIENTS**

Drug disposition of many drugs has been studied in obese patients, and some general conclusions can be drawn. Absorption of drugs evaluated to date is unchanged due to obesity. Apparent volume of distribution is greatly increased for some drugs, including most benzodiazepines, phenytoin, verapamil, and lidocaine. Modest increases in volume of distribution have been noted for methylxanthines, aminoglycosides, vancomycin, ibuprofen, prednisolone, and heparin. Distribution of digoxin, cimetidine, and procainamide is unchanged in obesity. The mechanism for the increased distribution of some drugs and unchanged distribution of others in obesity is unclear. It may be due in part to the lipophilic character of the drug molecule; however, other complex and as yet poorly understood factors contribute to the variability in drug distribution in obese patients.

Protein binding of drugs bound to albumin is not dramatically changed in obesity. In contrast, some studies report that drugs bound to AAG may have increased binding related to increased serum AAG concentration; however, this is not a consistent finding.

Oxidative drug biotransformation is minimally changed in obesity with the exceptions of ibuprofen and prednisolone, for which clearance increases as a highly correlated function of total body weight. In studies of paracetamol (acetaminophen), lorazepam, and oxazepam, drug conjugation uniformly increased as a function of body weight in obesity. Drug acetylation may be unchanged in obesity; however, only procainamide has been evaluated thus far. High clearance drugs, including lignocaine, verapamil, and midazolam, demonstrate no change in clearance in obese individuals compared with normal body weight controls. Renal clearance of drugs is little changed for some drugs evaluated (digoxin, cimetidine) and increased for others (aminoglycosides, unmetabolized procainamide).

V. POSITIVE DRUG INTERACTIONS

Not all drug interactions are undesirable, and some drug interactions are used strategically to enhance clinical effect. Positive drug interactions are classified as follows:

1. **Additive:** The resultant pharmacologic effect is equivalent to the combined effect of each drug used alone. An example of an additive interaction is the use of dopaminergic and anticholinergic drugs in the treatment of parkinsonism.

2. **Synergistic:** The effect produced is greater than the sum of the effects of each drug used alone. The antimicrobial combination of sulfamethoxazole and trimethoprim to block two sites in the folic acid meta-

bolic pathway in microorganisms exemplifies this type of interaction. Some consider synergism in fact only additive.

3. **Augmentative:** One drug induces and prolongs increased concentration of another drug in a body fluid. Probenecid has this effect on penicillin, and carbidopa on levadopa.

4. **Necessary/facilitative:** Both drugs are needed for the effect or one drug makes it possible for the other to produce its desirable action. This type of interaction is exemplified by the combined use of penicillin and an aminoglycoside to treat enterococcal infections.

5. **Reparative:** One drug counteracts the undesireable effects of another. Combining the laxative effect of magnesium hydroxide with the constipating effect of aluminum hydroxide produces an acid-neutralizing effect while sometimes avoiding adverse consequences on the gut.

6. **Complementary:** Drugs are combined that act through different physiologic mechanisms to produce a common beneficial clinical effect. The treatment of congestive heart failure with both digitalis glycosides and diuretics illustrates this mechanism.

VI. ANTACIDS

1. **Decreased absorption of tetracyclines:** Because of possible formation of nonabsorbable complexes and/or increase in intragastric pH, patients should be advised not to take antacids within 3 to 4 hours of taking tetracycline. Concurrent administration with enteric-coated tablets may cause the enteric coating to dissolve too rapidly, resulting in gastric or duodenal irritation.

2. **Decreased absorption with ketoconazole:** Alkalinization of the urine may shift the elimination kinetics of some antibiotics, possibly leading to crystalluria and nephrotoxicity.

VII. ANTIBIOTICS

1. **Penicillins:** Varied degree of protein binding, which should be considered in patients taking multiple drugs. Can interact with aminoglycosides and reduce the half-life and serum concentrations, especially in patients with impaired renal function.

2. **Erythromycin:** High degree of protein binding. Can inhibit carbamazepine metabolism, resulting in increased plasma concentrations. Can increase cyclosporine plasma concentrations. Increased prothrombin time with increased risk of bleeding in patients taking warfarin. Decreases the biotransformation of theophylline, possibly increasing side effects. Can enhance the hypoglycemic effect of oral hypoglycemic drugs. Can increase digoxin serum level.

3. **Tetracyclines:** Patients intolerant to lidocaine may be intolerant of oxytetracycline, and those intolerant of procaine may be intolerant of tetracycline. Long-term use may result in reduced contraceptive reliability for oral estrogen-containing contraceptives. Tetracyclines may partially counteract the anticoagulant effect of heparin. Concurrent use with magnesium-containing laxative may result in the formation of nonabsorbable complexes.

VIII. ANTIDEPRESSANTS

Antidepressants generally are highly protein bound, and this should be considered in patients taking multiple drugs. Sedative effects of doxepin (Sinequan) and possibly other tricyclic antidepressants may be potentiated with propoxyphene by inhibiting hepatic metabolism. Use with sympathomimetic drugs may potentiate cardiovascular effects, possibly resulting in arrhythmia, tachycardia, or severe hypertension or hyperpyrexia. Use with monoamine oxidase (MAO) inhibitors may result in an increased incidence of hyperpyretic episodes, convulsions, hypertensive crisis, and even death. The peripheral antimuscarinic effects of tricyclic antidepressants may decrease or inhibit salivary flow, especially in the elderly. Extrapyramidal reactions may result in increased motor activity of the head, face, and neck. Blood dyscrasia effects may result in increased incidence of oral microbial infections, delayed healing, and gingival bleeding.

IX. CARDIOVASCULAR DRUGS

1. **Digitalis:** Low protein binding for digoxin and high protein binding for digitoxin should be considered in the patient's medical history. Metabolism of digi-

toxin may be accelerated by drugs that induce microsomal enzymes, including phenylbutazone, phenobarbital, phenytoin, and rifampin; the magnitude of this effect is variable among patients. Untoward effect of dental interest is neuralgic pain, usually involving the lower third of the face and simulating trigeminal neuralgia, which may be the earliest, most severe, and even the sole manifestation of digitalis intoxication.

2. **β-Adrenergic blocking agents:** Antihypertensive effects may be reduced when used concurrently with nonsteroidal anti-inflammatory drugs (NSAIDs), possibly as a result of inhibition of renal prostaglandin synthesis and sodium and fluid retention caused by the NSAIDs, especially indomethacin. Use with sympathomimetic agents with α- and β-adrenergic effects (e.g., epinephrine) may result in increased α-adrenergic activity with the risk for hypertension and excessive bradycardia. With multiple injections of lidocaine, β-adrenergic blockers may slow hepatic metabolism and possibly increase the risk of lidocaine toxicity.

X. H₂ RECEPTOR ANTAGONISTS

1. **Cimetidine, ranitidine:** The degree of protein binding of these drugs generally is low. By increasing gastric pH, they have the potential to affect the bioavailability of medications whose absorption is pH-dependent. H_2 receptor antagonists may prevent the degradation of acid-labile drugs. These drugs also have the ability to inhibit the hepatic microsomal drug metabolism system, possibly affecting the elimination of other medications that require hepatic metabolism.

XI. NONSTEROIDAL ANTI-INFLAMMATORY ANALGESICS

In general, these drugs have a very high degree of protein binding, which should be considered when other drugs are present. Patients intolerant of one of the NSAIDS, including aspirin, may be intolerant of any of the others. NSAIDS may cause bronchoconstriction or anaphylaxis in aspirin-sensitive asthmatic patients, especially those with the triad of aspirin intolerance, asthma, and nasal polyps. NSAIDS inhibit platelet aggregation; however, their antiplatlet effect, unlike that of aspirin, is reversible. Prolonged concurrent use of acetaminophen with an NSAID may increase the risk of adverse renal effects. NSAIDS, especially indomethacin, may decrease lithium renal clearance, resulting in increased serum lithium concentration. NSAIDS may increase the hypoglycemic effect of antidiabetic agents, because prostaglandins are directly involved in the regulatory mechanisms of glucose metabolism and possibly because of displacement of the oral antidiabetic agents from serum proteins. Concurrent use of two or more NSAIDS may increase the incidence of gastrointestinal side effects, including ulceration or hemorrhage. Aspirin can increase the serum level of methotrexate.

XII. OPIOID (NARCOTIC) ANALGESICS

Narcotic analgesics have a low to high degree of protein binding, which should be considered when other drugs are present. Opioid analgesics may decrease salivary flow and may cause discomfort, especially in patients with dentures. Geriatric patients may be more susceptible to the effects, especially the respiratory depressant effects. Geriatric patients may metabolize or eliminate these medications more slowly than younger adults, and lower doses or longer dosing intervals should be considered. Meperidine can interact with MAO inhibitors and cause an unpredictable, severe, and sometimes fatal reaction, including immediate excitation, sweating, rigidity, severe hypertension or hypotension, respiratory depression, seizures, hyperpyrexia, and cardiovascular collapse. Meperidine is contraindicated in patients who have received an MAO inhibitor within 14 to 21 days. There is increased risk of orthostatic hypotension in patients taking antihypertensive medication. Tobacco smoking may increase the metabolism of propoxyphene. Chronic use of phenytoin and rifampin may increase methadone metabolism.

BIBLIOGRAPHY

Abernethy DR, Greenblatt DJ: Drug disposition in obese humans: An update. *Clin Pharmacokinet* 1986; 11:199–213.

Caranasos GJ, Stewart RB, Cluff LE: Clinically desirable drug interactions. *Ann Rev Pharmacol Toxicol* 1985; 25:67–95.

Drug Information for the Health Care Professional. Rockville, Md, US Pharmacopeial Convention, 1990.

Garattini S: Drug metabolism and actions in the aged. *Drug Nutrient Interact* 1985; 4:87–97.

Wood M: Plasma drug binding: Implications for anesthesiologists. *Anesth Analg* 1986; 65:786–804.

Prescriptions and Prescription Writing

Lorraine B. Tesch

This chapter addresses the generalities of prescription writing, the use of generic vs. trade name prescriptions, guidelines for the use of controlled substances, and the use of placebos.

I. PRESCRIPTION WRITING
A. Prescription sections
1. **Superscription:** General background information regarding the dentist (name, address, telephone number) and the patient (name, address, age) and the date the prescription is written.
2. **Inscription:** Specific information regarding the drug (generic or proprietary name, or both) and the dosage.
3. **Subscription:** Directions to the pharmacist for filling the inscription (number of capsules or tablets to be dispensed or the volume of liquid), the number of refills allowed and time constraints, direc-

253

tions to be listed on the container label, and for a controlled substance the DEA number.

4. **Transcription:** Instructions to the patient, to be listed on the container label.

5. **Signature and educational degree of prescribing doctor:** A signature is required by law only for certain controlled substances (schedule II drugs). This law allows other prescriptions to be phoned in by the doctor to the pharmacist when necessary.

B. **Guidelines for prescription writing**

1. Simply because a patient perceives that he or she has not received adequate attention unless a prescription is written is insufficient reason to write one.

2. Obtain an accurate and complete patient history, including whether the patient is taking any drugs prescribed by other doctors or any over-the-counter drugs; both can affect the dosage or effects of the drug being prescribed.

3. Use a separate prescription blank for each drug ordered. Avoid using prescription blanks with trade names printed on them. Never presign a prescription blank, and always store blank prescription pads in a secure place.

4. Write out numbers rather than using digits so that the prescription cannot be altered.

5. Prescribe sufficient drug and at adequate dosing intervals to maintain therapeutic blood level. PRN is not sufficient for drug dosage.

6. Review the manufacturer's data for prescription drugs; changes are made periodically that affect indications for use, dosage, or side effects.

7. Specify whether and how many times the prescription may be refilled. PRN is not appropriate.

8. Keep a record of all drugs prescribed for each patient.

9. Instructions listed on the drug container for the patient to follow must be specific. Patient understanding as to how to take the prescribed medication varies. Patient noncompliance ranges between 20% and 60%. Full disclosure is verbally given

regarding the prescription before the patient leaves the office. Stress the need to consume all of the prescribed medication, as in the taking of antibiotics, even if the patient is feeling better before the prescribed amount is taken.

10. Instructions regarding anticipated side effects as well as the use of alcohol while taking the prescribed drug should be explained to the patient verbally. Advise the patient to call the office should side effects develop. Clarification of the dosing schedule may be necessary. If the medication prescribed is to be taken q6h, explain that this means every 6 hours in a 24-hour period, not four times a day while awake, between breakfast and bedtime.

11. Cost factors should be considered when prescribing medication, especially in the elderly. The choice of prescribing a generic vs. a trade name drug is based on professional experience and current data on the particular medication. Although the active portion of the formulation of a generic drug is required by law to be the same as in the proprietary drug, inert substances may differ and thus affect absorption, distribution, and elimination rates. These factors will depend upon the substances and the manufacturing processes.

C. **Prescriptions for infants and children**
   Infants and children can be grouped as follows:
   1. Neonates.
   2. Infants 30 days to 2½ years of age.
   3. Children 2½ years to adulthood.
      Individual drugs are prescribed on the basis of milligrams per kilogram body weight. **Never exceed the maximum adult dosage.**

II. CONTROLLED SUBSTANCES
The Controlled Substance Act places drugs of abuse in one of five categories: schedules I, II, III, IV, and V. The schedule in which a drug is placed depends on its medical usefulness, its potential for abuse, and the degree to which the drug may lead to psychologic or physical dependence.

Schedule I: Drugs that have no acceptable medical use and high risk for abuse (e.g., LSD, mescaline, peyote, heroin, marijuana, and THC [tetrahydrocannabinol]).

Schedule II: Drugs with an accepted medical use but high potential for abuse (e.g., meperidine HCl [Demerol], hydromorphone HCl [Dilaudid], codeine, morphine, amphetamines, acetaminophen–oxycodone HCl [Percocet], aspirin–oxycodone HCl [Percodan], and short-acting barbiturates.

Schedule III: Drugs with a medically accepted use and low to moderate potential for abuse (e.g., drug mixtures containing specified, limited, quantities of codeine with either aspirin or acetaminophen, and nonnarcotic drugs).

Schedule IV: Medically acceptable drugs with low potential for abuse and low risk for dependence (e.g., flurazepam HCl [Dalmane], diazepam [Valium], chlordiazeporide HCl, [Librium], propoxyphene [Darvon], pentazocine [Talwin], and chloral hydrate.

Schedule V: Mixtures of drugs containing low quantities of narcotics, such as a codeine cough preparation, with relatively low potential for abuse and risk for dependence.

Any clinician who prescribes, administers, or dispenses a controlled substance must comply with the guidelines stated in the Controlled Substance, Drug, and Device and Cosmetic Act, Section 4. The minimum requirements are that the doctor be board licensed and prescribe, administer, or dispense in good faith in the course of professional practice and within the treatment principles of the patient-doctor relationship as deemed acceptable by the profession. On prescribing, administering, or dispensing a controlled substance a written record on the patient's chart is made and retained for a minimum of 5 years following the date of the last entry in the record. The information should contain: (1) name, quantity, and strength of the controlled substance, (2) date of issuance, (3) directions for use, and reason for issuing the controlled substance. A schedule II substance may be ordered by telephone only in an emergency, and must be followed by a written prescription delivered to the pharmacy within 72 hours. Prescriptions listed under this schedule are deemed nonrefillable. Schedule III, IV, and V drugs may be ordered by telephone or in writing and may be renewed if specified on the prescription. Prescriptions may be renewed a maximum of five times within 6 months after the date of issue. The amount prescribed should not exceed the total needed to produce a minimum toxic effect if taken all at once. In addition, a separate prescription blank is suggested for each controlled substance prescribed.

III. PLACEBOS

The term "placebo" is derived from the Latin *placere,* "I shall please." Placebos are described as drugs used for their psychologic or psychophysiologic effect. This intended effect is unknown to the patient, and may be unknown to the therapist as well. Placebos have nonspecific effects against the condition for which they are given. Such conditions may include any type of medicine (active, nonactive, topical, parenteral), surgical procedure, mechanical procedure, or psychotherapy.

A large number of medical textbooks in various specialities (including pharmacologic textbooks) merely mention placebos in the experimental role. Subjectively, placebos have been shown to relieve anxiety, depression, chronic headache, postoperative pain, and myofascial pain dysfunction. Measureable effects of placebo action include change in pupil diameter, alteration in blood pressure, change in serum lipoprotein, eosinophil, and lymphocyte counts, and changes in serum electrolyte and steroid levels. The placebo effect has been proposed to be a combination of physiologic and psychologic interactions. The placebo, as studied by Beecher, exerts its action on the processing of pain by the CNS. In addition, the placebo effect is more effective when stress level is high. If a patient anticipates pain relief, a positive placebo response takes place. Another hypothesis regarding the placebo effect is its initiation of impulses originating in the cerebral cortex. These impulses may be further stimulated by positive verbal suggestions regarding the "drug" that may act on the cortex, and through autonomic pathways, neural channels, and humoral mechanisms can mediate physical changes without the patient's awareness.

The placebo effect is not imaginary nor suggestive in the usual sense of the word. Adverse reactions caused by a placebo are unpredictable and vary from patient to patient. Toxic symptoms include drowsiness, vertigo, headache, depression, insomnia, and gastrointestinal disturbances. There have been reports of hallucinations following withdrawal of a placebo supposed to have addictive properties, if the patient is led to believe the "drug" is in fact addictive. Further, placebos given to healthy volunteers who believed they were receiving an active drug experienced side effects similar to those experienced by the active drug taker.

Outside the realm of clinical trials, the questions of when and by what means placebos should be prescribed in general practice continue to persist. In this setting it is perceived that the usefulness of a placebo may be destroyed if informed consent is sought, because the success of the placebo is assumed to depend on the patient's ignorance and suggestibility. It has further been assumed that since the placebo is relatively harmless and can be beneficial, the lack of informed consent cannot possibly matter.

Increased medical costs may occur due to additional expenses following the use of placebo in place of well-established therapy when use of the placebo fails. Clinicians may be pressured into prescribing placebos by patients eager for cures and instant alleviation of symptoms. Conversely, the patient who discovers that an inert substance has been taken may lose faith in the medical profession and subsequently refuse to take medication that could be vital to recovery.

Placebos are regarded as trivial and quite outside the realm of ethical evaluation. However, placebos are not trivial.

The prohibition of the administration of placebos should not be absolute, however. Each case needs to be carefully evaluated to ascertain if the benefit greatly outweighs the possible harm. The following guidelines have been suggested:

1. Placebos should be used only after careful diagnosis.
2. Only inert, and not active placebos should be used.
3. No outright lie should be told the patient, and questions should be answered honestly.

4. Placebos should never be given to patients who have asked not to receive them.
5. Placebos should not be used when other treatment is clearly called for or when all possible alternatives have not been weighed.

BIBLIOGRAPHY

Beecher HK: Ethics and clinical research. *N Engl J Med* 1966; 274:1354–1360.

Bok S: The ethics of giving placebos. *Sci Am* 1974; 231:17–23.

Newman MG, Goodman AD: *Guide to Antibiotic Use in Dental Practice*. Chicago, Quintessence Publishing Co, 1984, pp 162–173.

Prescribing Controlled Drugs. *Dent Med Dig* 1987; 9:1–6.

Safe, Effective and Therapeutically Equivalent Prescription Drugs, ed 7. State of New York Department of Health, 1988.

Stout KW: *Prescription Writing and Therapeutics in Dental Practice*. Philadelphia, Kenneth W Stout, 1986.

Chapter 15 _____

Antibiotics, Analgesics, and Other Prescribed Drugs

Lorraine B. Tesch
Raymond F. Zambito

_____

I. ANTIBIOTIC AGENTS

The normal flora of the oral cavity includes approximately 300 morphologically and biochemically distinct bacterial groups or species. Under normal conditions a wide variety of both aerobic and anaerobic microorganisms grow in the regions of the tongue, gingival crevice, oropharynx, dental pulp, and plaque. Although the quality and quantity of flora vary at different oral areas, the anaerobes equal or outnumber the aerobes at all sites. These microorganisms are nonpathogenic and part of the normal oral flora until there is a breach in the host defense mechanism.

When this mechanism breaks down there is a need to either kill the offending organisms or prevent them from proliferating. This is accomplished through the use of antibiotics, debridement, or both.

Antibiotics are organic substances, either produced by microorganisms or synthetically manufactured, that have the ability, in low concentrations, to destroy or inhibit growth of bacteria and other microorganisms. Antibiotics are most effective in patients with an intact immune system. Control of the microorganisms occurs when the microorganisms have been decreased to a level at which the immune system can be effective. The actions of antibiotics are highly selective, acting specifically against aspects of bacterial metabolism but usually not against those of tissue cells. Antibiotics are usually administered systemically, with relatively few side effects that are often unrelated to the nature of their antibacterial activity.

The clinician should try to differentiate a bacterial from a viral infection before initiating therapy, because antibiotics are ineffective against viruses. Obtain a clear history from the patient.

In general, antibiotics are prescribed when clinical features of infection are present, such as red and tender edema of the affected oral area that does not appear to be resolving spontaneously. Fever is an important sign of significant infection. Fever, by definition, is elevation of temperature 1 degree or more above normal (37.0° C, 98.6° F), although many infectious disease experts consider a temperature of 38.0° C (100.5° F) indicative of fever. In addition, the patient's circadian rhythm may alter the temperature level.

Rationale for therapy is based on four major considerations:

1. Clearly established need for antibiotics.
2. Careful patient history regarding previous antibiotic use and experience, including self-medication.
3. Laboratory susceptibility studies.
4. Knowledge of the side effects of antibiotic or sulfonamide to be prescribed.

Prophylactic and therapeutic distinctions are important:
1. **Prophylaxis:** Prevention begins **preoperatively** and continues for up to 24 hours.

2. **Therapeutic:** An established infection exists. Thus higher doses of drug are prescribed and the antibiotic is prescribed for a longer period. Duration of therapy depends on site of infection, clinical response, and knowledge of the bacteria responsible for the infection. In usual circumstances the antibiotic is prescribed for 7 to 10 days. For example, streptococcal infections require potassium phenoxymethyl penicillin (Pen-Vee-K) administered for 10 to 14 days with follow-up visits every 48 to 72 hours. Antibiotic therapy should continue for 48 hours beyond the remission of *all* symptoms of infection.

Cultures should be performed to determine the offending organism. Dental infections are caused by mixed anaerobic and aerobic bacteria, predominantly streptococci or staphylococci. Choice of empiric therapy after initial cultures may be based on a detailed history and the clinical presentation, especially in the presence of fever.

Studies performed during the last two decades have demonstrated the pathologic role of anaerobic bacteria in odontogenic infections. In the past, the majority of infections were reported as aerobic, principally as *Staphylococcus* and *Streptococcus*. Recent reports reveal mixed aerobic-anaerobic infections, with anaerobes outnumbering aerobes. Previous methods of specimen collection and culture did not preserve anaerobic bacteria; thus they were not adequately isolated and identified (see Moenning et al, 1989).

Sabiston et al. (1976) reported on 65 dental abscesses. Of 58 (65.9%) specimens, on average 3.8 distinct species were isolated from each culture. Likewise, Kannangara et al. (1980) studied 61 dental infections and found that 74% were due to either mixed aerobic-anaerobic or exclusively anaerobic infections. On average, 2.6 anaerobic microorganisms were isolated from each infection. Aderhold et al. (1981) studied 50 dental abscesses and found 96% of the specimens to be anaerobic in origin. Sixty-eight percent were mixed aerobic-anaerobic microorganisms, and 28% were anaerobic. The most common aerobic organisms were α-hemolytic streptococci; no staphylococci were identified. The authors concluded, and their findings concur with those of Sims (1974), that a high percentage of staphylococci were contaminants. This low proportion of staphylococci in dental infections was confirmed by other investigators.

Penicillin may not be effective in patients with penicillin-resistant organisms in the oral flora, for example, alcoholic patients, those with insulin-dependent diabetes (type II), hospitalized patients, and those who have received antibiotic therapy recently. Altered flora can cause a dramatic change in penicillin susceptibility, from 98% to 40%–50% for anaerobes and from 85% to 70% for aerobes.

Guidelines for Prescribing Antibiotics

1. Identify the offending organism.
2. Consider the pharmacology as well as the toxicity of the drug chosen.
3. Attempt to limit treatment to one antimicrobial agent rather than combination therapy. This can be achieved by prescribing either a broad-spectrum antibiotic or one that interferes with the synergism of the offending bacterium.
4. Consider tissue penetration.

Prescription of antibiotic therapy presupposes knowledge of:

1. Which antibiotic to prescribe.
2. How much to prescribe in a loading dose.
3. How much to prescribe in a maintenance dose.
4. How many days the antibiotic should be taken.
5. Which route of administration to use (PO, IM, IV).

Before prescribing any medication, the clinician should read the FDA-approved package inserts for complete drug information. If the infection is severe or life-threatening, the drug of choice should be bacteriocidal rather than bacterostatic, and administered parenterally. Bacteriocidal properties cause a reduction in the microorganisms, whereas bacteriostatic antibiotics simply inhibit bacterial growth while allowing the host's immune system to combat the remainder of the offending microorganisms.

The mechanisms of antimicrobial action vary with the antibiotic and its site of antibacterial activity.

Antibiotics that interfere with cell-wall synthesis include:

- Penicillins
- Cephalosporins
- Cycloserine
- Vancomycin
- Bacitracin
- Amphotericin

Human cells do not possess cell walls; thus these antibiotics attack the bacteria without interfering with normal physiology and cellular chemistries.

Antibiotics that interfere with intracellular protein synthesis include:

- Chloramphenicol
- Tetracyclines
- Kanamycin
- Neomycin
- Gentamycin
- Streptomycin
- Macrolide antibiotics (erythromycin, troleandomycin)

Antibiotics that affect cell membrane (detergent effect) include:

- Polymyxins
- Colistin
- Novobiocin
- Polyene antifungal agents (nystatin, amphotericin)

Antibiotics that affect nucleic acid metabolism include:

- Griseofulvin

Antibiotics that affect intermediary metabolism include:
- Sulfonamides
- Isoniazid, aminosalicyclic acid, ethambutol

Antibiotics that affect DNA synthesis include:

- Quinolones (nalidixic acid, norfloxacin, ciprofloxacin, ofloxacin)

Principles of Antibiotic Therapy

1. Antibiotics are more effective against acute than chronic infections.
2. Penicillin is the antibiotic of first choice in dentistry. Use adequate dosage for adequate duration.
3. Clindamycin or erythromycin is the antibiotic of second choice, especially in patients allergic to penicillin.
4. Depending on the organism, its site, and severity of infection, systemic administration is preferred to topical; oral administration is preferred to injection except in severe infections.
5. A clinical response should be noted in less than 48 hours.
6. If possible, cultures should be taken before beginning antibiotic therapy.
7. Multiple antibiotic therapy should be avoided.
8. Antibiotics are not effective against viruses or fungi. Specific antiviral and antifungal agents may be administered in these cases.
9. Broad-spectrum antibiotics may be indicated.

A. Penicillins

Systemically administered penicillins are found in exudate from acutely inflamed tissue. They are effective in the treatment of acute ulcerative gingivitis. Penicillins are more effective in treating acute infections than chronic infections. Penicillin G is highly effective against most oral gram-positive and negative cocci, such as non-penicillinase-producing staphylococci, streptococci, and pneumococci, but fewer gonococci. *Treponema pallidum, Actinomyces,* and *Clostridia* are susceptible to penicillin.

The most frequently used antimicrobial agents are the penicillins, because of their clinical efficiency, minimal toxicity, low cost, and spectrum of activity. Penicillins are bacterio-cidal and act principally, although not exclusively, by inter-fering with cell wall synthesis. The family of penicillins consists of:

1. **Penicillin G**
   a. **Crystalline penicillin G sodium**
   b. **Penicillin G procaine** (benzylpenicillin procaine) (benzathine benzylpenicillin)
   c. **Penicillin G benzathine**
2. **Penicillin V** (phenoxymethyl penicillin, phenethicillin, propicillin, phenbenicillin)
3. **Extended-spectrum penicillins**
   a. Aminopenicillins (ampicillin, amoxicillin)
4. **Antipseudomonal penicillins**
   a. Carboxy penicillins (carbenicillin, ticarcillin)
   b. Ureidopenicillins (azlocillin, mezlocillin, piperacil-lin)
5. **Semisynthetic (antistaphylococcal) penicillins**
   a. Methicillin
   b. Nafcillin
   c. Isoxazolyl penicillins (oxacillin, cloxacillin, diclox-acillin; flucloxacillin not available in the United States)

NOTE: Penicillin should not be prescribed with tetracycline; these drugs antagonize each other's antibacterial activity. If the compliant patient does not respond within 48 hours to the peni-cillin prescribed, drainage of the abscess and/or administration of another antibiotic should be considered.

The following interactions hold for both penicillin G and V:

1. Inactivated by fruit juices.
2. Absorption inhibited by food or antacids.
3. Antagonized by some other antibiotics and rendered useless.
4. Excretion inhibited by probenacid (Benamid).

Because of their long history of efficacy, both penicillin G and penicillin V often are considered the standard by which other antibiotics are judged for the treatment of odontogenic in-fections.

1. **Penicillin G**
   Penicillin G was one of the first penicillins in general
   use. The most effective route of administration of penicillin G is intravenously. The oral form of penicillin G
   is no longer used because it is destroyed by gastric
   acid. Penicillin G has a narrow spectrum, which may
   be advantageous because it renders superinfection (due
   to widespread destruction of the mucosal flora) less
   likely. Bacteria such as *Streptococcus pyogenes, Streptococcus pneumoniae,* viridans streptococci, anaerobic
   gram-positive cocci, gram-negative bacilli, and spirochetes are susceptible to penicillin G.
   a. **Crystalline penicillin G sodium**
      In a patient with a severe odontogenic infection,
      crystalline penicillin G is administered intrave-
      nously, and hospitalization is required. Penicillin G
      can be administered over long periods without seri-
      ous side effects.
   b. **Penicillin G procaine**
      Penicillin G procaine (benzylpenicillin procaine) has
      the same antibacterial spectrum as penicillin G. Its
      route of administration is exclusively intramuscular.
      It is inappropriate for use in most odontogenic in-
      fections.
   c. **Penicillin G benzathine**
      The suggested use for penicillin benzathine is pro-
      phylaxis against rheumatic fever. It is administered
      intramuscularly monthly because it attains a low
      serum level for prolonged periods (15 to 30 days).
      Penicillin benzathine is recommended for the treat-
      ment of early syphilis and syphilis of more than 1
      year's duration, excluding neurosyphilis.
2. **Penicillin V** (phenoxymethyl penicillin)
   The activity of penicillin V is similar to that of penicillin G. Because this form of penicillin is acid stable, it
   is orally administered and readily absorbed in the gut.
   It is recommended that the drug be taken before meals
   for maximum effectiveness. Serum levels as high as
   those with penicillin G cannot be readily obtained
   with penicillin V. Efficacy of penicillin V depends partially on patient compliance. Oral administration is cho-

sen in compliant patients with mild to moderate infections.

The most serious complication of penicillin G or V therapy is the development of an allergic reaction. Penicillin allergy is known to occur in about 10% of the patient population, but effects usually are mild. The allergic reaction may be manifested by pruritic erythema, sometimes followed by accompanying fever and joint inflammation.

The most severe reaction caused by penicillin is anaphylactic shock. If the patient is highly allergic, the reaction is swift, within seconds to 2 hours after antibiotic administration, and may include any or all of the following: facial parasthesia, coldness of the hands and feet, wheezing due to bronchospasms, and edema of the face. In the most severe cases patients develop peripheral circulatory failure, accompanied by a rapid fall in blood pressure, resulting in pallor, sweating, coldness of the skin, a fast thready pulse, and loss of consciousness. Patients may asphyxiate from edema. Death can occur in moments if the reaction is not reversed. In general, the more rapid the onset of the allergic reaction the more severe it can be expected to be. Although severe anaphylaxis can occur with the administration of oral penicillin, the reaction is seen less frequently or may not develop as rapidly. The patient's previous history of reaction to penicillin is important; patients who develop anaphylactic reactions usually have experienced mild reactions in the past.

Patients with a history of allergies in general, such as hay fever, asthma, or eczema, are more likely to have an allergic reaction to penicillin. It is possible that patients will have taken penicillin without ill effect, then experience an anaphylactic reaction with subsequent penicillin use. Although the incidence of anaphylactic shock is low, it is recommended that penicillin not be administered to an atopic patient who is to undergo surgery with general anesthesia. This should not deter prescription of penicillin for dental infections in patients with no specific penicillin or β-lactam allergy history. Penicillin continues to be the drug of choice.

3. **Extended-spectrum penicillins**
   The aminopenicillins (ampicillin and amoxicillin) are extended-spectrum penicillins active against some gram-negative bacteria (e.g., *Haemophilus influenzae, Escherichia coli), Salmonella,* and *Shigella.* They are destroyed by gram-positive and gram-negative β-lactamases.
   a. **Ampicillin**
      Ampicillin is a bacteriocidal antibiotic. Because of its broad spectrum of activity, ampicillin is often prescribed empirically when treatment is initiated without the benefit of a precise bacteriologic diagnosis. The drug is acid stable and is adequately absorbed from the gastrointestinal tract, with a half-life of 1 to 1½ hours.
   b. **Amoxicillin**
      Amoxicillin has almost identical properties as ampicillin, and similar antibacterial properties. It is administered orally. One difference is that it is not useful in the treatment of susceptible *Shigella* infections. Serum levels of orally administered amoxicillin are twice as high as with orally administered ampicillin, and its absorption is less compromised with concomitant food intake.
         The risk for allergic reaction with the administration of ampicillin and amoxicillin is similar to that with penicillins G and V. Rash occurs more frequently. Neutropenia has been described with both ampicillin and amoxicillin. Diarrhea is less frequent with amoxicillin than with ampicillin. Even with large intravenous doses, ampicillin is rarely associated with renal toxicity or mild hepatotoxicity. Central nervous system toxicity is associated with large doses, especially in the presence of renal insufficiency.
4. **Antipseudomonal penicillins**
   a. **Carboxy penicillins** (Carbenicillin, Ticarcillin)
      (1) **Carbenicillin** is active against such organisms as *H. influenzae, Neisseria meningitidis, Neisseria gonorrhoeae,* and *E. coli; Salmonella, Clostridium, Lactobacillus, Actinomyces,* and *Propionibacterium* species; and *Arachnia propi-*

onica. This drug is not adequately absorbed from the gastrointestinal tract.

Adverse reactions include hypokalemia, dose-dependent prolongation of bleeding time, and allergic reactions. Oral indanyl carbenicillin is adequately absorbed from the intestinal tract, although serum levels are too low to treat infections other than simple urinary tract infections.

(2) **Ticarcillin** has similar pharmacokinetics and antimicrobial spectrum as carbenicillin, but is twice as active against *Pseudomonas aeruginosa*.

b. **Ureidopenicillins** (Azlocillin, Mezlocillin, Piperacillin)

These antibiotics are administered intravenously. They are excreted through the kidneys, and display dose-related pharmacokinetics. **Azlocillin** is at least eight times more active against *P. aeruginosa* than carbenicillin is. **Piperacillin** is as much as twice as active against *P. aeruginosa* as azlocillin is. **Mezlocillin** is effective against *Klebsiella* species.

Adverse reactions of azlocillin, mezlocillin, and piperacillin include platelet aggregation interference, neutropenia, hepatitis, and allergic reactions.

B. Other antibiotics

1. Cephalexin

Cephalexin is a broad-spectrum cephalosporin. However, it is not a first-line drug for odontogenic infections. The spectrum of this drug does not cover the predominant bacteria found in most dental infections. If susceptibility testing shows that the offending organism is within the antimicrobial spectrum of cephalexin, it may be used.

2. Clindamycin

Treatment with clindamycin produces excellent clinical results against serious gram-positive aerobic and anaerobic infections caused by *Staphylococcus, Pneumococcus, Bacteroides, Fusobacterium, Antinomyces, Eubacterium, Peptococcus, Peptostreptococcus*, and *Veillonella* species.

Clindamycin is the drug of choice in penicillin-allergic patients with serious odontogenic infections, and is recommended in patients with infection unresolved with penicillin therapy. Clindamycin's most serious reported side effect is pseudomembranous colitis due to colonization with toxin-producing *Clostridium difficile.*

3. **Erythromycin**

Erythromycin is recommended in patients with nonserious odontogenic infection who are allergic to penicillin.

4. **Tetracyclines**

The tetracyclines, for example, doxycycline, are recommended in patients allergic to penicillin who have nonserious infection. This drug has been effective against obligate anaerobes, but clinical studies have shown that some strains of bacteria develop resistance. Tetracycline is most effective when used for localized juvenile periodontitis. The most common side effect of this drug is development of a fungal overgrowth on mucous membranes (e.g., gastrointestinal tract, vagina).

There are few indications for use of tetracyclines in children younger than 8 years. The tetracyclines bind calcium salts and are incorporated into the bones and teeth when administered during calcification, resulting in permanent discoloration of the enamel and dentine. When affected teeth erupt, they may first appear yellow, but gradually change to gray, brown, or intermediate shades.

5. **Metronidazole**

Metronidazole is recommended in patients with serious anaerobic infection who are allergic to penicillin or in whom a serious anaerobic infection is unresolved with penicillin therapy. The spectrum of this drug is exclusively anaerobic: *Bacteroides fragilis, Clostridium* species, *Eubacterium* species, and *Peptococcus* species. The drug is not effective against aerobic organisms, including staphylococci and streptococci.

6. **Quinolones**

Quinolones are synthetic compounds that were introduced as urinary tract infection agents. Nalidixic acid was the first quinolone released (1964), but was only available as an oral agent, and its use was restricted to uncomplicated urinary tract infections without systemic complications. More recently, norfloxacin and ciprofloxicin have come into general use. Ofloxacin is soon to be released, and ciprofloxicin will soon be available for intravenous use in serious systemic infections.

The newer quinolones are active against *Enterobacteriaceae* and *Pseudomonas aeroginosa, H. influenzae, N. gonnorrhoeae,* various *Rickettsia, Legionella pneumophila,* staphylococci, streptococci, and other organisms. Quinolones are ineffective agents against anaerobic bacteria.

Because quinolones have no effective anaerobic spectrum, they are not considered primary agents for use in dentofacial infections or infections of odontogenic origin. Use in combination with an antibiotic (e.g., clindamycin or metronidazole) with an anaerobic spectrum must be considered when using this class of drugs for infections associated with the oral cavity.

C. **Antifungal agents**

A fungal infection can occur on the mucous membranes as the result of treatment with certain antibiotics and/or in a patient with impaired host defense mechanisms. The most common cause of oral fungal infection is *Candida albicans,* resulting in thrush, denture stomatitis, and several types of mucocutaneous candidosis.

1. **Nystatin** is only effective topically.
2. **Ketoconazole** is effective against oral esophageal candidiasis and a few other fungi.
3. **Fluconazole** is effective against mucocutaneous and deep-seated *Candida* and other fungal infections.

D. **Prophylactic antibiotic therapy**

Prophylactic antibiotic therapy is recommended by the American Heart Association for patients who are undergoing surgical procedures or instrumentation involving mucosal surfaces or contaminated tissue and are at risk for infective endocarditis or endarteritis. Inasmuch as it is not possible to predict in which patients these infections will develop, prophylactic therapy is recommended for those at-risk patients who are undergoing procedures likely to cause bacteremia, for example, routine dental examination if it will produce bleeding, periodontal probing, prophylaxis, and minor surgical procedures such as incision and debridement of abscesses. Prophylactic antibiotics are recommended for patients with prosthetic joints. The incidence of bacteremia is exacerbated in patients with gingival inflammation and periodontal disease. In addition, edentulous patients may develop bacteremia from ulcers caused by improperly fitted dentures.

Prophylaxis should be directed against those organisms commonly implicated in endocarditis following dental procedures, such as α-hemolytic streptococci. The theory of the development of endocarditis in susceptible patients proposes that the diseased cardiovascular structures develop areas of abnormal blood flow and high turbulence that results in bacterial colonization.

Cardiac conditions for which prophylactic antibiotic therapy is recommended include:

1. Prosthetic cardiac valves.
2. Most congenital cardiac malformations.
3. Surgically constructed systemic-pulmonary shunts.
4. Rheumatic valvular disease.
5. Acquired valvular dysfunction.
6. Idiopathic hypertropic subaortic stenosis.
7. Previous history of bacterial endocarditis.
8. Mitral valve prolapse.
9. Transvenous pacemakers.

This list is not all-inclusive. The practitioner must exercise clinical judgment based on clinical experience in determining the duration and choice of antibiotic when special circumstances apply. For example, prophylactic therapy is recommended in patients who do not have clinically detectable heart disease but have a documented previous episode of bacterial endocarditis.

The recommended standard antibiotic regimen of therapy for dental procedures that result in gingival bleeding and oral-respiratory tract surgery is as follows:

1. **Adults**
   a. **Oral regimen:** 3 gm amoxicillin VPO 1 hour before the procedure, followed by 1.5 gm amoxicillin VPO 6 hours after the initial dose.
   b. **Parenteral regimen:** In patients unable to take oral

TABLE 15–1.

Antibiotic Dosage Regimen (in Patients With Normal Renal Function)

		Dosage	
Drug	Route	Adult	Pediatric
Penicillins			
Crystalline penicillin G	IV	2 million units q2–4h as IV piggyback over 20 min	300,000–1.2 million units
Penicillin G benzathine	IM	1.2–2.4 million units, single injection	25,000–50,000 units/kg/day
Penicillin V	PO	250–500 mg, q6h	
Semisynthetic penicillins			
Nafcillin	IV	2 gm q4–6h	50–100 mg/kg/day
Oxacillin	IV	0.5–2 gm q4–6h	50–200 mg/kg/day
Cloxacillin	PO	250–500 mg q4–6h, before meals	25–50 mg/kg/day
Dicloxacillin	PO	250–500 mg q6h, before meals	25–50 mg/kg/day
Extended-spectrum penicillins			
Ampicillin	PO	250–1,000 mg q6h	50–400 mg/kg/day, depending on indication
	IV	1–2 gm q4–6h	

Drug	Route	Dose
Amoxicillin	PO	250–500 mg q8h	20–100 mg/kg/day, depending on indication
Carbenicillin	IV	30 gm/day in 6 divided doses	400–600 mg/kg/day
Ticarcillin	IV	4–18 gm/day	50–300 mg/kg/day
Azlocillin	IV	4–18 gm/day	
Mezlocillin	IV	4–18 gm/day	
Piperacillin	IV	4–18 gm/day	
Other antibiotics			
Cephalexin	PO	0.5–2 gm q6h	25–50 mg/kg/day
Clindamycin	PO	150–600 mg q6h	8–20 mg/kg/day divided q6–8h
	IV	600 mg q6h or 900 mg q8h	
Erythromycin	PO	250 mg q6h	30–50 mg/kg/day, divided doses
		500 mg, q6h	
	IV	2–4 gm/day	
Tetracyclines	PO, IV	1–2 gm in 4 equal doses, depending on severity of infection	Not recommended in children ≤9 yr
Doxycycline	PO, IV	200 mg on day 1, then 100 mg/day	Not recommended in children ≤9 yr
Metronidazole	PO	500 mg q6h	
	IV	500 mg–1 gm IV q6h	
Ciprofloxacin	PO	500–750 mg bid	
	IV	200 or 400 mg q12h	

amoxicillin, 2 gm ampicillin IV or IM 30 minutes prior to the procedure and 1 gm IV or IM 6 hours after the initial dose.

For patients allergic to amoxicillin, the following regimen is recommended by the American Heart Association:

a. **Oral regimen:** Erythromycin 1 gm PO 2 hours before the procedure, then 500 mg PO 6 hours after the initial dose.

b. **Parenteral regimen:** Clindamycin 300 mg IV 30 minutes before the procedure, and 150 mg 6 hours after the initial dose.

2. **Children**

a. **Oral regimen:** Amoxicillin 50 mg/kg 1 hour before the procedure and 25 mg/kg 6 hours after the initial dose. (Not to exceed the adult dose).

b. **Parenteral regimen:** For children unable to take oral amoxicillin, ampicillin 50 mg/kg IV or IM 30 minutes before the procedure and 25 mg/kg 6 hours after the initial dose.

For children allergic to amoxicillin:

a. **Oral regimen:** Erythromycin 20 mg/kg 2 hours before the procedure, and 10 mg/kg 6 hours after the initial dose.

b. **Parenteral regimen:** Clindamycin 10 mg/kg IV 30 minutes before the procedure, and 5 mg/kg 6 hours after the initial dose.

Table 15–1 gives the dosage regimen for the various antibiotics.

II. ANALGESIC AGENTS

Pain management in the dental patient is individualized according to the quality of the pain, its severity, cause, and chronicity. Pain arises when there is a noxious stimulus to the tissue as the result of destruction or injury. Such trauma can occur by means of a disease process, formation of an abscess, or through surgical intervention or extraction of a tooth. Biochemical mediators stimulate the pain process by release of histamine, bradykinin, prostaglandins, and other short-acting substances.

Prostaglandins (PGs) are naturally occurring substances composed of fatty acids found throughout body tissues. Addition of a letter to the abbreviation (e.g., PGD, PGE, PGF, PGG, PGH) is used to differentiate variations in the basic prostaglandin molecular structure. The actions of the prostaglandins and their related compounds are broad and variable, and affect many organ systems. The precursor of this substance in humans is arachidonic acid. Arachidonic acid has important effects on the immunologic, inflammatory, and hypersensitivity processes. It stimulates the inflammatory-immunologic response by producing erythema, increased local blood flow, increased vascular permeability, and edema. Four general groups of drugs inhibit the action of arachidonic acid:

1. Inhibitors of arachidonic release; these inhibit synthesis of products distal to this step (e.g., corticosteroids).
2. Inhibitors of the steps between arachidonic acid release and PGH formation (e.g., classic nonsteroidal anti-inflammatory agents, aspirin, indomethecin).
3. Inhibitors acting distal to PGH formation.
4. Inhibitors of non-PGH pathways.

Prostaglandins sensitize the receptors to respond to an acknowledged pain mediator, bradykinin, therefore contributing to the analgesic effect of the prostaglandin inhibitors.

Dental pain is best managed by selecting a pharmacologic agent from one of the three widely used groups:

1. **Local anesthetics** are used parenterally or topically. They block nerve impulses that originate at the peripheral site of pain, preventing the impulses from reaching the brain, where they would be interpreted as pain.
2. **Peripherally acting analgesics** inhibit the release of the biochemical mediators that produce pain at the site of injury. In addition to their analgesic properties, the majority of these drugs are anti-inflammatory and antipyretic.
3. **Narcotics and opiates** act on the central nervous system. They effect the interpretation of and reaction to impulses that reach the brain. There is no activity from

these agents at the site of the injury or on nerve conduction.

When selecting the proper analgesic, the degree of analgesia sought, potency, minimal adverse potential, and desired effect, including anti-inflammatory effect, must be considered.

A. Analgesics

A class of drugs that inhibit the synthesis of PGs is the nonsteroidal anti-inflammatory drugs (NSAIDS). NSAIDS are aspirin-like in that they have antipyretic activity. In addition, NSAIDS reduce or eliminate the production of sensitizers for peripheral nerve endings associated with pain. They also appear to have a ceiling effect for analgesia; further dose increments did not lead to increased analgesia when headache was used as a pain model. Therapeutic as well as side effects of NSAIDS are proposed to be the result of inhibition of PG synthesis. Side effects particular to an individual NSAID can also be due to other than PG synthesis inhibition.

Side effects of NSAIDS include:
1. **Gastrointestinal:** gastritis, possible ulcer formation.
2. **Central nervous system:** confusion in the elderly, headache.
3. **Blood clotting:** increased bleeding time, interaction with anticoagulants.
4. **Renal effect:** renal failure leading to hypertension or congestive heart failure.
5. **Hepatic effect:** in rare cases, may cause an increase in transaminase concentrations.

The severity of side effects from NSAIDS parallel their ability to inhibit PG synthesis. NSAIDS may be recommended for mild to moderate pain.

Approximately 16 NSAIDS are available at this writing, and at least 20 more are undergoing clinical trial. Their idiosyncratic differences in effectiveness and toxicity, many of which cannot be explained, are the reason for the number of NSAIDS. Possible conditions that effect the differences are hydrophilicity or lipophilicity of the drug, ionic charge, and genetic regulation of receptor sites. One definitive indication for selecting an NSAID and dose is a patient older than 75 years. Older patients have less than half the nephrons of patients 30 years of age; therefore, drugs with a longer half-life may reach levels of analgesia before aspirin and other salicylates.

1. **Aspirin and other salicylates**

    Aspirin and its analogues are the most widely used analgesic for dental pain. In addition to its analgesic properties, the anti-inflammatory and antipyretic properties of such compounds are useful, respectively, in reducing edema and fever that may follow oral surgery. Salicylates have the capacity to inhibit cyclooxygenase and the production of prostaglandins. Because of the inhibition of cyclooxygenase, platelets cannot produce thromboxane, which is the first step in blood clotting. This can be detrimental in patients scheduled for surgery. Aspirin acetylates the platelets, and it takes 7 to 10 days for the body to manufacture new platelets. Bleeding time can be prolonged for up to 1 week; thus aspirin should not be used in presurgical dosing for its analgesic effect. On the other hand, there is recent evidence that a dose of one aspirin daily can prevent myocardial infarction and/or cerebrovascular accident due to clots initiated by the same mechanism.

    When aspirin alone is ineffective for pain and the pain migrates toward the moderate end of the scale, it is recommended that its analgesic properties be enhanced by combining aspirin with another drug, such as codeine. Aspirin has a ceiling effect; that is, no additional analgesic effect is gained after 15 grains are taken.

    The side effects of aspirin and its analogues include tinnitus, dizziness, and loss of hearing. These symptoms arise from doses much higher than therapeutic doses. Depending on the dosage, especially with doses higher than the daily recommendation, side effects may include nausea, vomiting, gastrointestinal bleeding, stimulation of the respiratory system followed by depression, disruption of the acid-base balance and water-electrolyte balance, vasomotor paralysis, and a uricosuric effect. Patients with a history of allergies may be hypersensitive to aspirin, often displayed by urticaria, bronchospasms, laryngeal edema, and hypotension. In arthritic patients, the suggested daily limit of aspirin is 6 to 8 gm.

2. **Propionic acids**

This is the largest class of drugs that are both anti-inflammatory and analgesic. They are metabolized in the liver and excreted in the urine. The analgesic effect of these drugs is equal, but they have varying times of absorption to achieve peak plasma levels. Examples include:

- Naproxen (Naprosyn)
- Ibuprofen (Motrin, Rufen, Advil, Nuprin)
- Ketoprofen (Orudis)
- Fenoprofen Ca (Nalfon)

3. **Indoleacetic Acids**

This group of drugs are metabolized in the liver and excreted in the urine. Sulindac has a greater tendency to produce diarrhea because of the potential for these drugs to biliary secretion and a small bowel–liver circulation. Drugs in this group include:

- Indomethacin (Indocin)
- Sulindac (Clinoril)
- Tolmetin (Tolectin)

4. **Fenamic Acids**

These drugs have a relatively high degree of toxicity and are not recommended for more than 7 consecutive days in adults. A common side effect is diarrhea and blood dyscrasias, with prolonged use. Examples:

- Mefenamic acid (Ponstel)
- Meclofenamic acid (Meclomen)

5. **Oxicam**

This group is represented by one drug, piroxicam (Feldene). Because of its long elimination half-life, allowing once-a-day dosage, it is recommended chiefly as an antiarthritic. Its dose and duration of action as an analgesic have not yet been fully determined.

6. **Phenylbutazone** (included for the sake of completion)
This group is represented only by Butazolidin. Because of its severe toxicity, it is recommended only when other NSAIDS fail. As a result of sodium-retaining properties, it may cause hypertension and add to existing headache. Serious bone marrow, hepatic, and renal toxicity has been associated with phenylbutazone, more so than with other NSAIDS.

7. **Acetaminophen**
Although acetaminophen is not an NSAID, it does have analgesic and antipyretic properties. It has little effect as an anti-inflammatory agent, possibly because of the particular cyclooxygenase enzymes that act on the PGs involved in inflammation, which differ from those cyclooxygenase enzymes that act on PGs dealing with pain and fever. It might also be for these reasons that acetaminophen has little or no effect on the gastrointestinal tract, bleeding time, or uric acid excretion.

Acetaminophen has the following advantages over narcotic analgesics:

a. It is not subject to DEA control.
b. It usually does not depress the CNS, which permits the patient to be fully amublatory and functional.
c. It does not produce tolerance or dependence.

In large doses, this group of drugs can cause serious hepatotoxicity. Drugs in this group include:

- Tylenol
- Datril

Either aspirin or acetaminophen alone is recommended to treat mild to moderate dental pain. When inflammation is present postoperatively, aspirin is the better choice, because of acetaminophen's anti-inflammatory effect. The anti-inflammatory effect occurs at two to three times the analgesic dose. In patients allergic to aspirin, acetaminophen is the drug of choice. Be aware of patients with aspirin hypersensitivity when prescribing NSAIDS, because of the possibility of cross-allergy. When either of these two drugs is used in adults for postoperative dental pain, the dose recommended is 975 mg, rather than the more common 650 mg, providing no medical reasons preclude the increased dose. Studies have shown that acetaminophen has more analgesic activity at the higher dose. The recommended dose of acetaminophen in pediatric patients varies with age and weight (Table 15–2). Aspirin is not recommended in pediatric patients, because of the risk for Reye syndrome.

A narcotic analgesic is prescribed for moderate to severe pain. An opioid may be prescribed when pain relief is not obtained from one of the milder, nonopioid analgesics. The smallest dose that provides relief of pain should be prescribed, because increasing dosage may be required to maintain an analgesic effect over a long period. Physiologic addiction to opioids takes at least 2 weeks to develop. Short-term administration is recommended. The side effects of opioids involve various body systems. Central nervous system effects include sedation, alteration of mood, euphoria, constriction of pupils, and nausea and vomiting. Respiratory depression may occur, and is dose related. Effects on the cardiovascular system by central mechanisms include vasodilation, orthostatic hypotension, and circulatory collapse. In the gastrointestinal tract, opioids decrease propulsive peristalsis in the small and large intestines and increase smooth muscle and sphincter tone. Side effects involving the genitourinary tract include increased ureter, bladder, and sphincter tone. Allergic reactions are rare, but may include urticaria, rash, and anaphylaxis.

8. Morphine

Morphine is a strong opiate when administered by injection. When taken orally, it has a high first-pass effect. This drug is associated with the development of tolerance (increased dosage is required to achieve the same level of analgesia) and addiction. It is recom-

TABLE 15-2.
Analgesic Dosage Regimen

Drug	Route	Dosage*	
		Adult*	Pediatric
NSAIDS			
Aspirin	PO	325–650 mg q4h	2–4 yr: 160 mg q4h
			4–6 yr: 240 mg q4h
			6–9 yr: 320 mg q4h
			9–11 yr: 400 mg q4h
			11–12 yr: 480 mg q4h
Propionic acid			
Naproxen (Naprosyn)	PO	250–500 mg bid	10 mg/kg bid
Ibuprofen (Motrin, Rufen, Advil, Nuprin)	PO	300–800 mg tid-qid	Not established
Ketoprofen (Oradis)	PO	150–200 mg/day in 3–4 divided doses	Not established
	Rectal	100 mg bid	
Fenoprofen (Nalfon)	PO	300–600 mg tid-qid	Not established
Indoleacetic acid			
Indomethacin (Indocin)	PO	25–50 mg bid-qid	1.5–2.5 mg/kg tid-qid } 1st 2 days
	Rectal IV	50 mg qid	1.5–2.5 mg/kg tid-qid
			2–7 days: 0.2 mg/kg at 12–24 hr intervals
			≥7 days: 0.2 mg/kg at 12–24 hr intervals
Sulindoc (Clinaril)	PO	150–200 mg q12h	Not established
Tolmetin (Tolectin)	PO	400 mg tid	≤2 yr: not established
			≥2 yr: 15–30 mg/kg/day in divided doses

(Continued.)

TABLE 15-2 (cont.).
Analgesic Dosage Regimen

Drug	Route	Adult*	Dosage* Pediatric
Fenamic acid			
Meclofenamic acid (Meclomin)	PO	200–400 mg/day in 3–4 divided doses	Not established
Mefenamic acid (Ponstel)	PO	250 mg q6h	Not established
Phenylbutazone			
Phenylbutazone (Butazolidin)	PO	Initial: 100–200 mg tid Maintenance: 100 mg/d-qid	Not recommended
Oxicam			
Piroxicam (Feldene, Butazolidin)	PO	10 mg bid	Not established
Acetaminophen (Tylenol, Datril)	PO	325–650 mg q4h	≤3 mo: 40 mg q4–6h
			4–12 mo: 80 mg q4–6h
			1–2 yr: 120 mg q4–6h
			2–4 yr: 160 mg q4–6h
			4–6 yr: 240 mg q4–6h
			6–9 yr: 320 mg q4–6h
			9–11 yr: 400 mg q4–6h
			11–12 yr: 480 mg q4–6h
Centrally acting analgesics: Opiates			
Morphine	PO	10–30 mg q4h	Individualized by physician
	IM, SC	5–20 mg q4h	100–200 mg/kg q4h
	IV	4–10 mg diluted in	50–100 mg/kg
		4–5 mL water for injection	
	Rectal	10–30 mg q4–6h	Individualized by physician

Drug	Route	Adult dose	Pediatric dose
Meperidine (Demerol)	PO	50–150 mg q3–4h	1.1–1.76 mg/kg q3–4h
	IM, SC	50–150 mg q3–4h	1.1–1.76 mg/kg q3–4h
	IV	15–35 mg/hr	
Hydromorphone (Dilaudid)	PO	2 mg q3–6h	Individualized by physician
	IM, SC, IV	2 mg q3–6h	Individualized by physician
	Rectal	3 mg q4–8h	Not established
Oxycodone (available only in mixtures)			
Oxycodone + acetaminophen (Tylox, Percocet)	PO	q4–6h	Not established
Oxycodone + aspirin (Percodan)	PO	q4–6h	≤6 yr: Not established
	PO		6–12 yr: ¼ half-strength tablet q6h
			≥12 yr: ½ half-strength tablet q6h
Codeine	PO	15–60 mg q3–6h	500 mg/kg qid
	IM, SC, IV	15–60 mg q4–6h	
	IM, SC		500 mg/kg q6–6h
Propoxyphene (e.g., Darvon)	PO	65–100 mg q4h	Not established
Agonists/antagonists			
Pentazocine (Talwin)	IM, SC, IV	30 mg q3–4h	Not established
Nalbuphine (Nubain)	IM, SC, IV	10 mg q3–6h	Not established
Butorphanol (Stadol)	IM	1–4 mg q3–4h	Not established
	IV	500 mg q3–4h	Not established
Tricyclic antidepressants			
Amitryptiline (Elavil)	PO	25 mg bid-qid	≤12 yr: not established
			Adolescent: 10 mg tid, 20 mg hs
Doxepin (Sinequan)	IM	20–30 mg qid	Not established
	PO	25 mg tid	Not established
Cyclobenzaprine (Flexeril)	PO	20–40 mg in 2–4 divided doses	Not established

*Analgesic doses given; anti-inflammatory dosage usually is twice the analgesic dose.

mended for use in severe pain not controlled by milder, less addicting agents.

9. **Meperidine**

   Meperidine (Demerol) is recommended in cases of severe pain. Prolonged use produces increasing concentrations of normeperidine, the first metabolite of meperidine, which has a longer half-life than the parent compound. Meperidine can cause CNS excitation, and at times grand mal seizures. It has been known to increase intracranial pressure. Twice the parenteral dose is required for an oral dose to have an equal analgesic effect.

10. **Hydromorphone and Oxycodone**

    These are potent oral medications, because they are completely absorbed. Oxycodone is available only in combination with either aspirin (Percodan) or acetaminophen (Percocet). Hydromorphone (Dilaudid) given orally is about five times less potent than the parenteral preparation.

11. **Codeine**

    Codeine is a commonly used analgesic, most often prescribed in combination with acetaminophen (i.e., acetaminophen with codeine phosphate tablets no. 3, which contain 30 mg codeine). Considered a weak opiate, codeine may be prescribed over a long period. Some authorities claim that it is impossible to induce addiction to oral codeine in doses clinically used to treat mild or acute pain. Codeine is metabolized in the liver to morphine, which is the active agent.

12. **Propoxyphene**

    Propoxyphene (e.g., Darvon) is a weak opiate. It is a mild analgesic with side effects similar to those of codeine. Overdosage can occur with various degrees of severity, leading to fluctuation between coma and convulsions, accompanied by cardiac and respiratory depression. Propoxyphene napsylate is the most effective form.

13. **Agonists/antagonists**

    These compounds have been shown to cause less respiratory depression and are less likely to be abused than the agonist opiates. They have a tendency to cause dysphoria, which has discouraged their use as an analgesic. These compounds are used when first-line drugs are ineffective. Some examples are:

- Pentazocine (Talwin)
- Nalbuphine (Nubain)
- Butorphanol (Stadol)

14. Tricyclic antidepressants

These drugs have most recently been used in treating chronic pain syndromes. The hypothesis for this particular use is an amplification of an inhibitory descending neural pathway that interacts with the incoming pain signal at the level of the spinal cord and has its origin in the parathalamic area with interconnections at the periaqueductal gray area. The descending pathways use serotonin and cathecholamines as neurotransmitters. The tricyclic drugs prevent the reuptake of serotonin from the neural clefts at nerve-axon junctions, thereby increasing the effect of serotonin. The incoming pain signal is suppressed and the neuronal segment located at the dorsal gray area of the spinal cord, thereby inhibiting its function of recognizing pain.

Side effects of this group of drugs include dry mouth, blurred vision, cardiac arrhythmias, constipation, and difficulty in urination. Serious side effects are urinary retention and glaucoma. Examples of tricyclic antidepressants are:

- Amitryptyline (Elavil)
- doxepin (Sinequan)

III. SEDATIVE/HYPNOTIC AGENTS

The sedatives and hypnotics are drugs whose action depresses the CNS; therefore they are used in the treatment of insomnia and anxiety. The sedative action produces drowsiness, calmness, and decreased motor activity. The hypnotic effect produces a state of unconsciousness similar to natural sleep. Loss of effectiveness of sedatives/hypnotics occurs in a relatively short period, and therefore their use should be limited. There is a potential for psychologic and physiologic dependence. Interactions may occur with the use of alcohol or other CNS depressants.

Benzodiazepines (diazepam [Valium] and chlordiazepoxide, mainly) are the prototypical drugs for today's practice. It is imperative that the correct metabolite of diazepam be chosen, and the need for such a sedative drug. The barbiturates are no longer considered drugs of choice unless otherwise indicated.

It is important to know which of the benzodiazepines metabolize into active and inactive metabolites. The four known drugs with active metabolites are chlordiazepoxide, chlorazepate, diazepam, and prazepam. These metabolites concentrate in the brain and remain active longer than the parent drug. With a longer half-life, these can produce significant blood levels, and repeated doses will cause accumulations that will affect the patient's response and recovery. The two drugs with inactive metabolites are lorazepam and oxazepam. Diazepam is absorbed rapidly when taken orally, and reaches peak level in 1 hour. The plasma half-life of diazepam is 20 to 50 hours. The drug is stored in adipose tissue, offering a rapid decline in plasma levels, then in about 6 hours reentry into the plasma, with recurrence of drowsiness.

Barbiturates can be either long- or short-acting. Short-acting barbiturates, which are effective in 15 to 30 minutes and last up to 6 hours, are secobarbital (Seconal) and pentobarbital (Nembutal). The most common indication for their use is insomnia. These drugs have been replaced by the benzodiazepines for the current practice. Their use is based on their relative inexpensiveness, convenience of administration, and widely published safety and efficacy data. The barbiturates cause drowsiness and mental impairment as well as respiratory depression.

Skeletal muscle spasms are the result of disturbances of the motor area of the CNS. Drugs that relax these muscles include:

- Diazepam (Valium)
- Carisoprodol (Soma Compound)
- Methocarbamol (Robaxin)
- Chlorzoxazone plus acetaminophen (Parafon Forte)
- Cyclobenzaprine (Flexeril)

IV. ANTIHISTAMINES

Antihistamines have both sedative effect and antipruritic action. They are prescribed for either symptomatic or prophylactic treatment of allergic reactions. Examples of this group of drugs are:

- Diphenhydramine (Benadryl)
- Chlorpheniramine (Chlortrimeton)
- Chlorpheniramine (Teldrin)
- Promethazine (Phenergan)

V. VITAMINS

Therapeutic vitamins are necessary for health. Vitamins should be supplied via the daily diet. Well-defined vitamin deficiencies are rarely seen in western society, but still exist. Although we depend on nutritional support to sustain necessary vitamin balance, in certain situations vitamin supplementation may be necessary. Therapeutic vitamins may be prescribed during pregnancy or during dieting for weight loss. Suggested multivitamins include:

- Thera-combex
- Surbex-T Filmtab
- Becotin
- Myadec
- Theragran

Vitamins with fluoride are commonly prescribed for young children, depending on the fluoridation of the local water supply. Sixty years of study have proved that the addition of fluoride to water supply prevents the development of caries. The recommended daily dose of fluoride for children younger than 3 years is 0.5 mg, and in children older than 3 years is 1 mg. Fluoride usually is prescribed in combination with a multi-vitamin:

- Tri-Vi-Flor
- Poly-Vi-Flor

- Adeflor
- Vi-Penta

VI. ANTICHOLINERGICS

Anticholinergics sometimes are prescribed to suppress salivary and bronchial secretions prior to a dental procedure. Examples include:

- Atropine sulfate (Donnatal)
- Propantheline (Pro-Banthine)
- Methantheline (Banthine)
- Glycopyrrolate (Robinul)

BIBLIOGRAPHY
Antibiotics

Aderhold L, Knother H, Frankel G: The bacteriology of dentogenous pyrogenic infections. *Oral Surg* 1981; 52:583.

Bochner F, Carruthers G, Kampmann J, et al: *Handbook of Clinical Pharmacology,* ed 2. Boston, Little, Brown, 1983.

Causon RA, Spector RG: *Clinical Pharmacology in Dentistry,* ed 4. New York, Churchill Livingston, 1985.

Dajani AS, Bisno AL, Chung KJ, et al: Prevention of bacterial endocarditis: Recommendations by the American Heart Association. *JAMA* 1990; 264:2919–2922.

Headings DL (ed): *The Harriet Lane Handbook: A Manual for Pediatric House Officers.* Chicago, Year Book Medical Publishers, 1975.

Kannangara DW, Thadepalli H, McQuirter JL: Bacteriology and treatment of dental infections. *J Oral Surg* 1980; 50:103.

Moenning JE, Nelson CL, Kohler RB: The microbiology and chemotherapy of odontogenic infections. *J Oral Maxillofac Surg* 1989; 47:976–985.

Neu HC: *Antimicrobial Prescribing.* Princeton, NJ, Antimicrobial Prescribing, 1979.

Newman MG, Goodman AD (eds): *Guide to Antibiotic Use in Dental Practice*. Chicago, Quintessence Publishing, 1984.

Orland MJ, Saltman RD (eds): *Manual of Medical Therapeutics,* ed 25. Boston, Little, Brown, 1987.

Physician's Desk Reference, ed 44. Oradell, NJ, Medical Economics, 1990.

Sabiston CB, Grigsby SW, Segerstrom N: Bacterial study of pyogenic infections of dental origin. *Oral Surg* 1976; 41:430.

Shulman ST, Amren DP, Bisno AL, et al: Prevention of Bacterial Endocarditis: A Statement for Health Professionals by the Committee on Rheumatic Fever and Infective Endocarditis of the Council on Cardiovascular Disease in the Young. *Circulation* 1984; 70:1123A–1127A.

Sims W: The clinical bacteriology of purulent oral infections. *Br J Oral Surg* 1974; 12:1.

Stout KW: *Prescription Writing and Therapeutics in Dental Practice*. Philadelphia, Kenneth W Stout, 1986.

Zambito RF, Cleri DJ (eds): *Immunology and Infectious Diseases* of the Mouth, Head, and Neck. St Louis, Mosby–Year Book, 1991.

Analgesics

Bochner F, Carruthers G, Kampmann J, et al: *Handbook of Clinical Pharmacology,* ed 2. Boston, Little, Brown, 1983.

Causon RA, Spector RG: *Clinical Pharmacology in Dentistry,* ed 4. New York, Churchill Livingston, 1985.

Dionne RA: *Pharmacologic Strategies for Suppressive Postoperative Dental Pain*. Bethesda, Md, National Institute of Dental Research, National Institutes of Health.

Drug Information for the Health Care Provider. USP Dictionary of Drug Names, ed 6. Rockville, Md, United States Pharmacopeial Convention, 1986.

Inhibitors of the synthesis of prostaglandins. II. *Dent Med Digest* 1982; 4:1–3.

Johns Hopkins University: *The Harriet Lane Handbook: A Manual for Pediatric House Officers*. St Louis, Mosby–Year Book, 1990.

Kantor TG: The management of pain by pharmacological agents. *Clin J Pain* 1989; 5:121–123.

Orland MJ, Saltman RD (eds): *Manual of Medical Therapeutics,* ed 25. Boston, Little, Brown, 1987.

Physician's Desk Reference, ed 44. Oradell, NJ, Medical Economics, 1990.

Prescribing Controlled Drugs. *Dent Med Digest* 1987; 9:1–3.

Stout KW: *Prescription Writing and Therapeutics in Dental Practice.* Philadelphia, Kenneth W Stout, 1986.

Use of non-steroidal anti-inflammatory agents (NSAIA) in dentistry. III. *Dent Med Digest* 1982; 4:1–3.

Index